Practical Psychiatry
in Medicine

Practical Psychiatry in Medicine

John B. Imboden, M.D.
Psychiatrist-in-Chief
Sinai Hospital of Baltimore, Inc.
Baltimore, Maryland

Associate Professor of Psychiatry
Johns Hopkins University
Baltimore, Maryland

John Chapman Urbaitis, M.D.
Associate Chief of Psychiatry
Sinai Hospital of Baltimore, Inc.
Baltimore, Maryland

Assistant Professor of Psychiatry
Johns Hopkins University
Baltimore, Maryland

foreword by
A. McGehee Harvey, M.D.
Professor of Medicine
Johns Hopkins University
Baltimore, Maryland

APPLETON-CENTURY-CROFTS / New York

78 79 80 81 82 / 10 9 8 7 6 5 4 3 2 1

Prentice-Hall International, Inc., London
Prentice-Hall of Australia, Pty. Ltd., Sydney
Prentice-Hall of India Private Limited, New Delhi
Prentice-Hall of Japan, Inc., Tokyo
Prentice-Hall of Southeast Asia (Pte.) Ltd., Singapore
Whitehall Books Ltd., Wellington, New Zealand

Library of Congress Cataloging in Publication Data
Imboden, John B 1925-
    Practical psychiatry in medicine.

    Includes index.
    1. Psychiatry.   2. Medicine, Psychosomatic.
3. Physicians (General practice) I. Urbaitis,
John Chapman, 1941–   joint author. II. Title.
[DNLM: 1. General practice. 2. Mental disorders.
WM100 I32p]
RC454.4.I4   616.8'9   77-13861
ISBN 0-8385-7910-8

Text design: Natasha Sylvester
Cover design: Kristin Herzog

PRINTED IN THE UNITED STATES OF AMERICA

Contents

Preface

Family physicians and other medical practitioners are entrusted with the responsibility of providing broad, comprehensive care for their patients. Therefore, the practicing physician must be able to use and understand the basic information in all the medical specialties.

Psychiatry in the past 20 years has become an increasingly important part of medical practice. Psychopharmacology and advances in psychotherapy now offer specific, efficacious means for treatment of many emotional disorders. Because most psychiatric problems can now be alleviated, partially or completely, by proper treatment, it is essential that the physician be able to investigate, diagnose, and initiate management of his patients with psychiatric difficulties.

It has been said that the greatest single failure of modern medicine is the frequency of inadequate communication between patient and physician. This may contribute to the paradox that physicians seem to be the target of increasing public criticism even though their technical, clinical effectiveness is greater than at any time in history. We believe that the physician who knows psychiatry and applies its principles in his daily practice will pay careful attention to this issue of communication and to the humanistic as well as the technical features of medicine.

We hope that this volume will be of practical value to physicians interested in the psychiatric aspects of the practice of medicine.

Many people have provided the authors with encouragement and helpful advice. The original suggestion to write this book came from Richard J. Johns, a friend and deeply respected colleague, who also has been of considerable assistance to us in other endeavors. We appreciate the editorial encouragement and invaluable aid which Richard Lampert provided us. Mary Blair and William Diehl read portions of the manuscript and offered useful suggestions. We wish to express our thanks to Mrs. Nina James, whose untiring and careful work in preparing the manuscript is deeply appreciated.

Foreword

Over the past three quarters of a century there has been an increasing appreciation of the importance of psychiatry in the day-to-day practice of medicine. Richard Cabot was among the first to recognize the importance of Sigmund Freud's ideas for the medical practitioner. When Lewellys Barker succeeded William Osler as Professor of Medicine at Johns Hopkins in 1905 he created the first full-time research divisions in a Department of Medicine: chemical, biologic, and physiologic. He wanted to create a fourth, psychiatry-in-medicine, but sufficient funds were not available at that time. His idea was finally implemented in 1946. George Draper, a pioneer in this field when he joined the staff of the Presbyterian Hospital, is reported to have been the first to use the term *psychosomatic medicine*.

After World War II psychosomatic medicine became an active field of research and among many important contributions, Flanders Dunbar's monumental compilation of emotions and bodily changes was a significant landmark in this field of study. Among early notable investigators were Franz Alexander, Stanley Cobb, Harold Wolff, and Felix Deutsch.

Attaching importance to the fact that the physician practices psychiatry continuously is easy, but translating this idea effectively into the preparation of physicians for medical practice is more difficult. During the past few decades, leaders in the effort have included John Romano, George Engel, and Theodore Lidz, among others.

A further step is the provision of a practical monograph dealing with this subject in a clear and understandable way for the use of the physician. This volume written by John Imboden and John Chapman Urbaitis, who have had a broad experience in the teaching of psychosomatic medicine and as psychiatrists serving in a very practical way as consultants to physicians, will fill an important need.

This approach recognizes the essential problem-solving nature of medical practice and thus deals with the clinical entities as they present on a day-to-day basis to the physician. Although psychiatry is still a complex area of medical practice, disorders once crudely lumped together as insanity have now been differentiated and categorized. These disturbances of nature or disease, which produce clearly recognizable psychiatric illness, and the accumulating experience with drugs that influence cerebral function have encouraged the belief that we can look forward to important advances in our understanding and ability to manage mental disorders. Many persons other than psychiatrists will be increasingly involved in both individual and group psychotherapeutic procedures in the future. Physicians, including the family physician and the internist, will be more deeply concerned in the identification and management of emotionally ill patients whom they encounter in their practices. Thus the need for a monograph of this type is great and should find wide appeal for the many groups concerned with this area of medical practice.

A. McGehee Harvey, M.D.
Professor of Medicine
Johns Hopkins University
Baltimore, Maryland

Practical Psychiatry
in Medicine

PART I

INTRODUCTORY CONCEPTS

Chapter

1

Psychiatry as an Integral Part of Medical Practice

Psychologic Reactions to Illness
Incidence of Primary Emotional Disorders in Medical
      Practice
Influence of Psychologic Factors on Physiologic Processes
Application of Psychiatric Principles in Treatment and
      Management
Physician–Patient Relationship
Chemotherapy

Psychiatry is a specialty whose principles find application in all of the disciplines of clinical medicine. Indeed, psychiatry has such an integral relationship with general medicine that it is accurate to say that the question which confronts the practicing physician is not *whether* he incorporates psychiatry in his clinical work but *how deliberately* and *how well* he does so.

Over 35 years ago, a distinguished internist, Louis Hamman, expressed his concept of psychiatry and of how it relates to medicine in these words:

The physician studies and practices psychiatry continuously, even when he protests that he has not the least knowledge of formal psychiatry. It is the chief

3

instrument of his success, even though he may practice it unconsciously. Psychiatry is a discipline whose purpose it is to study and understand the function and influence of mental processes and emotional states in health and disease. These dominate our life and influence every other function of the body, as in turn they are influenced by every other function.[1]

These assertions are more than exhortations to the clinician to be mindful "that his patient is a person." Hamman's comments remind us, rather, that an appropriate application of the principles of psychiatry to the practice of medicine extends the diagnostic and therapeutic skills of the practicing physician.

In this chapter we will describe in broad terms some of the major areas in which psychiatry is of particular relevance to medical practice.

PSYCHOLOGIC REACTIONS TO ILLNESS

It is a general principle in medicine that many of the signs and symptoms of disease are manifestations of physiologic responses which represent attempts to cope with noxious agents or with alterations in the organism which may themselves be consequences of adaptive processes. The tachypnea, leukocytosis, and fever of pneumonia, the ventricular hypertrophy of long-standing hypertension, and the general malaise and weakness which lead to energy-conserving rest are commonplace examples of physiologic coping responses that comprise an important part of many clinical syndromes. Equally important, though often receiving only token recognition, are the psychologic adaptations to serious illness and concurrent life stresses; these coping reactions also constitute an important part of the whole clinical picture.

The critical nature of psychologic coping responses to physical illness is apparent when one reflects upon (1) the importance of the patient's initial registration of discomfort; (2) his ability to make a judgment that help is needed; (3) his efforts to reduce intolerable uncertainty by developing his own theories about what is wrong with himself; (4) his feelings about those persons to whom he has entrusted his care; (5) his reaction to the separations, losses, and other hardships occasioned by illness and treatment; (6) his reaction to the extreme passivity and dependence which may be an unavoidable part of the illness experience; and (7) his ability, during convalescence, to relinquish the sick role and to resume his customary functions at home and work.

In the following example, the patient had no difficulty with the first step, the registration of discomfort, but found himself temporarily in a quandary about the second step, that of judging the significance of his symptoms and of his need for medical attention.

The patient was a 26-year-old intern in a large teaching hospital. During his third month on the surgical service he noted the onset of persistent, severe fatigue which was present upon arising in the morning and became worse as the day went on. Within a day or two following the onset of the fatigue, he developed a more or less constant, generalized, moderately severe headache. The young physician attributed these symptoms to his arduous work schedule, sleep deficit, and the frequently stressful atmosphere in which he worked. Noting that his fellow interns also were "always tired" and that he himself had long tended to have tension headaches, he tried to disregard his symptoms. After two or three days of private misery the patient developed a cough productive of a small amount of rusty sputum. He noted the latter symptom with a feeling of relief for until then he had interpreted his symptoms as "just neurotic," ie, as meaning that he was not able to bear up under the work load as well as his colleagues. Armed with an acceptable (to him) somatic symptom, the patient sought medical attention and was all but delighted when informed that the x-ray supported the diagnosis of viral pneumonia and that bed rest was prescribed. The patient convalesced rapidly from what was a relatively mild illness and returned to work after a few days with both his lungs and his self-esteem fully restored.

It is not rare for patients to develop feelings and fantasies which interfere with the decision to seek medical help or to comply with the therapeutic regimen, or which result in other behavioral responses that seriously complicate the illness course and convalescence. On occasion, the patient's emotions and behavior arising from psychologic coping processes may even dominate the clinical situation and require just as careful diagnostic evaluation and management as do other aspects of the illness.

INCIDENCE OF PRIMARY EMOTIONAL DISORDERS IN MEDICAL PRACTICE

Family physicians probably see far more patients with primarily psychiatric disorders than do psychiatrists. In 1939 Hamman reported the results of his review of 500 consecutive patients who consulted him. Two hundred and seventy-two were males, 228 females, and 68 percent were in the age span from 30 to 60 years. He found that 33 percent of these patients "suffered solely or predominantly from functional disorders." By the latter, the author makes it clear that he is referring to conditions in which no "organic cause" at all was found or in which there were "minor organic lesions" which could not possibly explain the symptoms.[1]

Estimates of the incidence of psychologic difficulties as the primary basis of complaints in various medical outpatient clinics have varied considerably, depending in part upon the strictness of definition. In a review of the records of 1000 consecutive referrals to a diagnostic clinic, Kaufman and Bernstein found that in 69 percent of the patients, there was no evidence of organic disease and in 81.4 percent psychologic factors were at the basis of their complaints.[2] Lipowski, in reviewing various reports on the frequency of psychiatric morbidity in nonpsychiatric divisions of general hospitals, concluded that there is evidence that from 30 to 60 percent of inpatients and from 50 to 80 percent of outpatients suffer from a significant degree of "psychic distress or psychiatric illness."[3]

These are very sobering figures even if one accepts only the lower end of the range of estimates as valid. One cannot conclude from these data that every practicing physician must have the capability of engaging his patients in intensive psychotherapy, but one can conclude that the development of diagnostic acumen and management skill in relation to emotional disorders is at least as important as it is in relation to other kinds of illness. The primary physician has the task of identifying an existing psychiatric disorder and of determining whether he himself will undertake management or refer the patient to a psychiatrist.

INFLUENCE OF PSYCHOLOGIC FACTORS ON PHYSIOLOGIC PROCESSES

The emotional state of the human being may influence bodily function in health and disease in a number of ways. Perhaps the most obvious of these is that attitudes and emotions may lead to behavior which has a direct impact, favorable or unfavorable, upon the individual's physical well-being, eg, seeking or avoiding needed help, complying or not complying with the therapeutic regimen, exercising moderation or being excessive in eating and drinking, and attempting to salvage one's life versus attempting to end it.

Further, emotional arousal itself is a physiologic process involving central neural pathways which influence peripheral processes and are influenced by them. The most classic example of this is the peripheral effects of sympathetic-adrenal discharge that accompanies fear or severe anxiety. There are a number of functional disorders in which somatic symptoms are the immediate consequence of physiologic changes accompanying emotional states, some but not all of which are mediated by the autonomic nervous system.

An intriguing and controversial series of investigations has led to the development of the theory that, in ways not yet understood, psychic stress may contribute importantly to the etiology of certain diseases in which there is structural change or tissue damage, ie, the psychosomatic diseases. Historically prominent among these disorders are duodenal ulcer and ulcerative colitis. Methodologic difficulties in proving the role of psychologic factors in the causation and alleviation of these and other diseases postulated to be psychosomatic are enormous and have led to hotly debated, conflicting points of view. It is obviously important for the practicing physician to be aware of psychosomatic concepts regarding disease etiology and to form his own judgment about the utilization of these concepts in planning treatment and management.

APPLICATION OF PSYCHIATRIC PRINCIPLES IN TREATMENT AND MANAGEMENT

The psychiatric aspects of treatment and management of medical patients in whom emotional or behavioral problems constitute a significant component of the clinical picture are manifold. Here we will only briefly mention the potential therapeutic power of the physician–patient relationship and the significance to general medicine of recent advances in psychopharmacology.

PHYSICIAN–PATIENT RELATIONSHIP

It behooves the physician to be aware that he himself, apart from any drugs or procedures which he may administer, is potentially a therapeutic agent, an agent that is not without the possibility of adverse side effects. In fact, the physician to whom the seriously ill or worried patient comes for help is in a unique position to form a remarkably influential relationship with the patient. For example, experienced clinicians have repeatedly observed that frequently the patient seems convinced that his physician is extraordinarily kind, compassionate, understanding, and competent even though he may have had scarcely more than an hour or two in the physician's company! This interesting phenomenon, which in a general sense may be called "transference," merits our thoughtful consideration. Other manifestations of transference, some of not so positive a quality, are also seen. In any event, there are occasions when the physician may utilize his relationship with the patient quite deliberately in order to attain specific objectives or to help the patient to do so. In doing this it is helpful to have some understanding of the principles of human behavior and of their application in forging diagnostic and therapeutic approaches to specific emotional or behavioral components of the clinical problem.

CHEMOTHERAPY

The last 25 years have witnessed a remarkable proliferation of chemotherapeutic agents for the treatment of a wide variety of psychiatric disorders. There has also been a heartening tendency to assess the effectiveness of these agents through carefully designed, controlled clinical trials. The proper use of psychotherapeutic drugs requires an accurate grasp of the conditions for which they are indicated and, as with any class of potent agents, the physician must be well grounded in their basic pharmacologic properties.

In addition to its present clinical applications, psychopharmacology has stimulated intensive research into basic aspects of neurochemistry and neurophysiology which may eventually shed light not only upon the mechanism of action of drugs but also upon the pathogenesis of certain psychiatric disorders.

With the foregoing considerations in mind, the remainder of this book will deal with the basic features of human behavior and personality development, the psychiatric evaluation of the patient, psychologic reactions to physical illness and treatment, psychophysiologic disorders, some common emotional or behavioral problems encountered in medical practice, the major psychiatric disorders, and, finally, psychologic and psychopharmacologic aspects of treatment and management.

REFERENCES

1. Hamman L: The relationship of psychiatry to internal medicine. Ment Hyg 23:177, 1939
2. Kaufman MR, Bernstein S: A psychiatric evaluation of the problem patient. JAMA 163:108, 1957
3. Lipowski ZJ: Review of consultation psychiatry and psychosomatic medicine. II. Clinical aspects. Psychosom Med 29:201, 1967

Chapter
2

Coping Behavior:
An Overview

It is the purpose of this chapter to discuss certain general principles and features of human behavior. We will begin with an overview of some of the ways with which people cope with the challenges and stresses of life. We will then briefly sketch the development of human behavior from infancy through adolescence, describe some of the general themes and vicissitudes in the period from young adulthood to old age and, finally, delineate those features characteristic of psychologic health and maturity.

It is hoped that this chapter will provide a useful background to the clinician in his basic conceptualization of personality function, in his seeking to understand behavioral responses to medical illness, and in the psychologic aspect of medical evaluation and management.

SOME BASIC FEATURES OF HUMAN COPING RESPONSES

In common with lower animals, the human being responds to stimuli, whether the stimuli originate in the external environment or from within himself. An outstanding differentiating feature of man is that his behavior is much less predictable than that of lower animals. As a consequence of the enormous complexity of variables that intervene between stimulus and response, the repertoire of human responses is incomparably larger than that of the next most highly evolved species. From a neurophysiologic point of view, one could attempt to describe this "enormous complexity of variables" in terms of that portion of the neuronal network of the central nervous system that is interposed, in any given instance, between the involved afferent and efferent peripheral nerve fibers. As important as this is, however, one cannot at this time give a useful account of the variables of human responses in neurophysiologic terms. While the findings of neurophysiology and neurochemistry are becoming increasingly relevant to the practice of clinical psychiatry, it is nonetheless evident that to approach the subjective and behavioral responses of human beings from a strictly neurophysiologic point of view would be analogous to evaluating the "answers" of a computer by examining its circuitry rather than by scrutinizing the way in which it has been programmed.

APPROACH AND AVOIDANCE

Perhaps a commonplace example will illustrate the preceding point.

Mrs. S. discovers a nodule in her right breast. Her first response is one of alarm but not panic. She immediately mentions the discovery to her husband and the next morning, after a night of fitful sleep, telephones her physician, explains the situation to him, and is given an appointment.

Her neighbor, Mrs. J., makes a similar discovery. She too responds with a feeling of concern but says nothing to anyone. In the ensuing two months, her husband observes that she is more moody than usual and seems a bit distant and preoccupied. One evening he too discovers the lump in her breast and over her protestations that it is "nothing" insists that she see the family physician.

In general terms, one could say that Mrs. S. coped with the disturbing "stimulus" by the response of "approach" while her neighbor's response to the same stimulus was one of "avoidance." It is of interest that Aitken-Swan and Paterson in reviewing the histories of 2700 patients with carcinoma of the breast, cervix, skin, and mouth found that in 45 percent, three months or more elapsed between the initial appearance of symptoms and reporting to the physician. Many of the patients who delayed going to the physician apparently did so to avoid having their fears of cancer confirmed.[1,7]

To understand fully the difference in response to the discovery of a nodule of the breast shown by these two patients would probably require an indepth study of both individuals. However, it is likely that a not-so-extensive study would enable one to gain partial comprehension of their behavior. Let us confine our attention to Mrs. J. Her history indicates that she has a tendency to respond to all threatening situations by putting her head in the sand and hoping they will somehow go away. Therefore her response to the discovery of a nodule in her breast turns out to be characteristic, ie, it is a feature of her character if one defines the latter as being comprised of relatively enduring attitudes and patterns of behavior. Further, it is learned that at the age of 12, Mrs. J. lost her mother who died of cancer and, at the time of this tragedy, she overheard some veiled criticisms of the physicians. As a consequence, Mrs. J. developed a rather fatalistic notion about the treatability of cancer and was distrustful of physicians. She may even have felt destined to suffer the same fate as her mother because she had felt inexplicably guilty following her mother's death, as if she may have been to blame in some way. This earlier family experience had reinforced her tendency to disregard anything having to do with cancer, including televised admonitions concerning early detection and treatment.

It should be noted that our limited knowledge of Mrs. J. does not enable us to say that she has a psychiatric illness. It is true that she tends to avoid facing unpleasant realities, but she may not be afflicted with a constellation of symptoms that would warrant the diagnosis of a specific neurosis. In further conversations with Mrs. J. it may be learned that she herself was quite unaware of some of the forces that contributed to her behavior, such as the influence of the early loss of her mother upon her

11

feelings about herself. If this is the case, the interviewer may infer from the data available that this and other important determinants of the patient's behavior were *unconscious*.

FURTHER ELABORATION OF COPING RESPONSES

The term "coping" usually connotes a type of response by which the individual successfully deals with a problem or adapts himself to a situation. If, however, one includes in this term behavior which is partially successful in allaying or preventing the emergence of an unbearable feeling, such as anxiety, the well known defense mechanisms can be regarded as a category of coping responses.

In the normal paradigm, the individual "copes" with his environment (internal and external) by being alert to relevant cues. Perception of a problem or opportunity is followed by actively seeking more information about it and by assessing its significance through comparison of the present situation with related past experiences. This in turn arouses the person to adopt a course of action which he believes suitable to his ability, his situation, and his needs or goals. It is unlikely that anyone always responds to the manifold situations of life in this ideal manner. Defensive behavior, in which some aspect of reality is avoided, is used to some extent by all human beings at various times in their lives. There are a variety of ways by which people may avoid painful aspects of the external world or minimize anxiety engendered by intrapsychic conflict.[2,4]

Repression   Repression refers to the exclusion of feelings and ideas from conscious awareness. Repression is a basic defensive operation which may be supported by other defenses such as *conversion*.

A 30-year-old housewife complained of severe marital problems. She looked forward to the day when the younger of her two children would be old enough to begin school because at that point she would feel freer to separate from her husband. Understandably, she professed a strong determination to avoid becoming pregnant.

Three months after the initial visit, the patient reported that she had not menstruated for two months and was sure that she was pregnant. Having apparently "forgotten" the feelings expressed earlier, she stated that she was looking forward to having another baby. There was only one complication: she had recently developed numbness and weakness of both hands which, she stated, would prevent her from holding a baby.

Denial   Denial is a process in which the individual avoids awareness of some painful aspects of reality, such as severe loss, bodily illness, or associated feelings. Under some circumstances, partial denial may serve a useful purpose by giving the individual time to muster his resources and adapt to a difficult or traumatic situation.[5] Occasionally, an individual who is informed that he has a serious illness may not seem to be emotionally disturbed by the news, may efficiently tend to his affairs preparatory to entering the hospital, and only later show unmistakable evidence of apprehension and grief. On the other hand, in the case of Mrs. J., described above, the denial of the existence of the breast nodule was, of course, maladaptive.

Reaction Formation   Reaction formation occurs when the repression of a feeling or wish is bolstered by its replacement in conscious awareness with its opposite; the resulting behavior often strikes others as excessive or overdone. A common example is shown by the excessively polite person who may, however, unconsciously reveal his underlying hostility by being condescending.

Displacement   Feelings and attitudes toward one individual or event are directed toward another in displacement.

A 6-year-old boy showed little outward sign of grief following the sudden death of his father. Several months later he reacted to the accidental death of a friend's dog by crying and wailing as though he had lost someone very close to him.

Rationalization   More often than not, a given behavior is the outcome of more than one motivation. In rationalization, there is selective awareness of acceptable motivations and disavowal or unawareness of unacceptable ones. Thus a patient explains to the physician that he must postpone a needed diagnostic procedure because of prior commitments but does not acknowledge that he fears what the examination will show.

Projection   In projection, an attribute of the self, such as a feeling or impulse, is ascribed to the external world, usually to another person.

A surgeon, upon encountering a technical problem that taxes his skill, scolds the nurse-assistant for not knowing what instrument to hand him.

Regression   The individual adapts to a currently stressful situation by retreating to a mode of behavior characteristic of an earlier period of his life. Like all defenses, regression may serve a useful, adaptive purpose. For example, the regression that is virtually inevitable in seriously ill, hospitalized persons may facilitate acceptance of the therapeutic regimen. On the other hand, regression to behavior such as pouting, passivity, and demandingness is seriously maladaptive under many circumstances of adult life, although it is often rewarded by others who are involved with the regressively behaving person.

PERSONALITY DEVELOPMENT

Students of human behavior have long been intrigued not only by the variability of human responses to nearly identical "stimuli" but also by the fact that a given individual tends to repeat patterns of behavior as he goes through life. This is one of the observations that has led to extensive examination of early childhood experiences, since detailed study of behavior patterns often reveals that they are traceable to the earliest periods of life that the subject can recall.

INFANCY AND CHILDHOOD

There is little doubt that the long period of relative helplessness and dependency of the human infant is of profound psychologic significance. In the first months of life, the baby is utterly dependent for life-support upon the mother or her substitute. It is impossible to know what is going on in the mind of the preverbal infant, but it is known that all infants are by no means alike at birth. Some are relatively placid, sleep a lot, cry little, and adapt to an eating and sleeping schedule with ease. Others are noisy, very active, sleep less, and are more demanding. Still others are in between. These differences are among the innate, perhaps hereditary, features that play a role in personality development and which doubtlessly influence the way the mother responds to the infant.

At the beginning, the mother characteristically becomes involved with the infant in a love relationship which has a rather "narcissistic" coloring; the baby, which not so long ago was a part of her own body, continues to be felt as an extension of herself for awhile. She is exquisitely aware of when her baby is hungry, wet, or in pain. The initial relationship of the mother and infant is such an intimate and interdependent one that some authors have referred to it as "symbiotic" in that the well-being of both mother and child depend (in different ways) on their relationship with each other.

Separation and Individuation   As the infant develops and learns to sit up, crawl, walk, and acquires language, he slowly separates himself from the mother. This process of separation and individuation begins in the first year of life, and under normal circumstances progresses rapidly during the remainder of childhood.[6] During this period, the child can be described as incorporating countless experiences of being cared for and as drawing upon these experiences in learning to care for himself. With this in mind, it is apparent that normal maturation is thwarted by severe maternal neglect on the one hand and by excessive indulgence on the

14

other. Most mothers seem naturally to be attuned to their child's increasing autonomy and experience an intermingling of sadness and joy in fostering it.

To return to the very early stage of development, it may be noted that the infant demands and usually receives quick gratification of his needs. It is not surprising that as he becomes aware of the existence of persons (parents) who meet these needs, he perceives them as godlike, ie, omniscient, omnipotent, and good. It is also inevitable that he will, for a while, believe in the magic power of his own thoughts and wishes, because at one time in his life he had but to cry and his needs would be met. Further, in the normal course of events in which the child has repeatedly had the experience that "being good" brings rewards and the opposite brings punishment, he will come to feel that when something good or bad (such as illness) happens to him, it is because he has done or thought something to deserve it; and, in varying degrees, this feeling persists throughout life.

Oedipal Phase   In the course of time, the child progressively develops the ability to tolerate the postponement of gratification, to relinquish unfulfillable wishes, and increasingly to take care of himself. By the third or fourth year, he has sufficiently mastered certain functions, such as walking, so that he now begins to use these functions somewhat automatically for his own purposes: he walks in order to go somewhere as opposed to concentrating on taking steps and keeping his balance. As Erikson has remarked, he is in a position to take the initiative and does so.[3]

At this stage it is not uncommon for children of both sexes to wish to have an exclusive relationship with mother and later, or alternatingly, with father. The intensity of these "oedipal" strivings may in part be determined by constitutional factors and is certainly influenced by the parents' behavior. In any event, the wish to take father's place with mother or vice versa is one with which the child is deeply conflicted: he loves the rival parent and does not wish to lose him or her, he feels afraid of punishment for his bad wishes, and he feels hopelessly unqualified. At this stage of development, the child, at least for the time being, normally represses his impossible dreams and achieves an identification with his parent whom he both loves and envies. He internalizes aspects of them, their values and ideals, ie, he develops a conscience, an inner mechanism of approval and prohibition, and so no longer regulates his behavior just in terms of external response: he is now capable of feeling guilt as well as shame. Being in possession of an inner set of values, ideals, and prohibitions (which, to be sure, will continue to develop and be modified), the child is now in a better position to venture forth from the home to kindergarten and school.

EARLY SCHOOL YEARS

The span of years from about age six to puberty is a time which Freud referred to as the "latency" period in the sense that it is one in which sexual drives and interests, though by no means absent, are comparatively dormant. This is a period of life in which there is consolidation, modification, and broadening of coping skills which were developed in the preceding years. During these years the child is progressively given more opportunities and encouragement to cope with life outside of home: in the classroom, the playground, the neighborhood, overnight visits with friends, and eventually a few weeks at camp. His exposure to peers and teachers gives him important opportunities to confirm or correct his notions about values and about what the "world" expects of people which he had heretofore derived from his immediate family. Boys and girls of this period tend to associate predominantly with members of their own sex, having special friends or chums, forming clubs and having secrets but usually without the preoccupation with defiance of authority so common at a later stage.

During these years there is a remarkable display of interest in a wide variety of subjects. Hobbies are cultivated, sometimes several at a time, and are often pursued to considerable depth and with much industry before being dropped. Erikson has commented that this is a period in which the individual becomes acquainted with the technology of his culture.[3] He is learning how to get along in the world so he can eventually provide for himself and others. If the individual has a successful experience in the grade school period, his sense of confidence in himself is justifiably enhanced. On the other hand, if the youngster has encountered learning difficulties, or has had serious failures, or has been confronted with a hostile and prejudiced environment, he may develop a feeling of inferiority and/or a self-defeating attitude of cynicism.

ADOLESCENCE

This period, spanning the years from the onset of puberty to about the age of 21, is one in which the child becomes an adult. Although normal development during adolescence is not invariably accompanied by periods of considerable turbulence, it frequently is. For this reason the assessment of adolescent behavior as being normal or pathologic may be quite difficult, requiring considerable experience on the part of the interviewer and sometimes requiring repeated observations over a period of time. This is an important point because premature or unwarranted labeling of the adolescent may, in itself, have undesirable consequences.

In the "phallic" phase of development (age three to six years) the child manages the conflicts associated with strivings for an exclusive relationship with one or both parents by identification with them, by developing an inner set of ideals and prohibitions, and by repressing his oedipal desires. At the time of puberty, when sexual sensations and drives come to the fore along with the beginning development of secondary sexual characteristics, the repressed (but not yet relinquished) oedipal strivings are mobilized and arouse conflict and anxiety at puberty as they had done previously. The degree to which this poses a challenge to the boy or girl at puberty depends upon the intensity of the repressed oedipal wishes and the strength and speed of development of sexual urges.

In any event, it is to be expected that with the "awakening" of genital sexuality at puberty, the adolescent will shift his emotional and libidinal investment to persons other than members of his own family, ie, to teachers, coaches, youthful leaders at school or in the community, and to his peers of the same or opposite sex. The adolescent may reinforce his move away from his parents by developing an attitude of indifference toward them. If he has not yet made the move away from his parents, he may temporarily guard himself from the possible intrusion of sexuality into his affectionate ties to them by developing an oppositional attitude and by becoming resentful, rebellious, and debasing of them. He may also utilize his expanding intellectual abilities by attempting to deny sexual, bodily feelings and concentrating his attention on abstract issues relating to art, religion, philosophy, and various forms of idealism.

These phenomena of early adolescence, namely, the displacement of emotional investment away from the parents to others, the development of oppositional attitudes, and relatively heavy emphasis on things intellectual do not, of course, arise solely in response to the anxiety-generating conflicts associated with sexuality. They are also anticipatory manifestations of ever greater emancipation from the parents and the assumption of an adult role. Undoubtedly, the extreme, almost caricatured forms of "independence" in early adolescence arise in part because the adolescent himself is ambivalent about growing up. He experiences, from time to time, a regressive pull, a desire to be a child again, and part of his extreme behavior is in reaction to these feelings within himself.

During adolescence, the individual normally becomes increasingly able to form lasting and comfortable relationships outside the home, to integrate sexual feelings in his relationship with others, and develops enough confidence in his own ideas and ideals that he can once more relate with his parents without feeling threatened. At the end of adolescence or the beginning of adulthood, he has developed a relatively stable set of values and goals, a sense of who he is and of what he wants to do with his life (at least in general terms); that is, he has developed an identity of his own. This development is greatly facilitated by giving the adolescent recognition, in the sense of encouraging him to accept an appropriate degree of responsibility and independence, tempered by the judicious proffering of support, guidance, and tolerance when he yields to the "regressive pull" and temporarily reverts to childish behavior.

The psychologic problems of adolescence are too numerous and complex for us to do justice to them here and we will limit ourselves to a few general comments.

In making the critically important emotional move away from the parents in the early teens, the adolescent will be hampered if, for any reason, he fears rejection, especially by his peers. Anything which makes him "too different" may arouse such fear, such as being too bright, too dull, too fat, too skinny, or having some physical blemish such as acne. The physician does well to take seriously the teenager who presents himself or herself for help with acne, obesity, or any other difficulty which may become the nucleus of a serious psychosocial problem.

The adolescent will also have difficulty in achieving emancipation if he has sensed that his parents do not want him to grow up; in this instance, he is hampered not so much by fear as by guilt. This type of problem is particularly apt to occur if he or she is the youngest of the children, or if one of the parents has a neurotic need to keep the youngster dependent.

Failure to achieve an enduring sense of values, goals, and vocational or career direction by the time of young adulthood is sometimes referred to as identity diffusion or identity crisis. Grave emotional illness may first become manifest around the transition stages of puberty and the end of adolescence.

ADULTHOOD

In adulthood, people continue to learn, change, and grow though usually not as rapidly or as dramatically as during childhood or adolescence.

With the successful denouement of adolescence, the young adult settles into or is clearly on a path toward careers of vocation, marriage, parenthood, or all three. In settling into a vocational career the healthy young person chooses his life's work for himself, though, to be sure, his choice is partially determined by identifications he has made with the significant other people in his life and he is doubtlessly influenced by encouragements or warnings that have come his way. In making his career choice, the young person attempts to match his own interests and aptitudes, as he assesses them, with the opportunities for training and for obtaining work which he believes are available to him. He must attain the technical competence required by his chosen field and must have the interpersonal skills necessary to form relatively lasting and productive relationships with superiors, peers, and underlings. It is not at all uncommon for the young adult to feel a certain amount of insecurity or anxiety at this stage of life because he has not yet had enough experience to be confident that his own abilities (as he assesses them) are sufficient for him to "make it" out in the world. The anxiety arising from a sense of disparity between his self-image, or what he is, and his image of what he ought to be may at times lead the young adult to withdraw or retreat from challenging situations on the one hand or, at the other extreme, to develop a defensive exaggeration of his abilities; but usually these swings in attitude are not as marked as those of adolescence. This type of concern is one of the factors related to the observation that neuroses, which are characterized by anxiety or symptomatic defenses against anxiety, often have their onset in young adulthood.

Most young adults get married and have children. Successful marriage requires the individual to have a capacity for intimacy with another person. Persons involved in an intimate relationship have enough trust in each other and enough confidence in themselves to reveal their feelings and needs while at the same time respecting each other's autonomy and privacy. Conflicts between the demands of work and those of the family are not uncommon and when they occur both parties of the marriage are called upon to order their priorities in a practical and flexible way.

Those young adults who marry and raise children have the enlightening experience of piloting someone else through the channels they themselves have traversed in the not-so-distant past. In doing so, the young parents are apt to encounter issues, problems, and conflicts in their children which are reminiscent of their own experiences at various stages of development. In parenthood, young adults not only give where they once received, and are depended upon, but also develop new dependencies on each other and their children which are not altogether unlike those from which they were previously "emancipated" through earlier waves of separation and individuation.

Most young adults have, to some degree, an illusion of indestructibility and an understandable feeling of having an abundance of time in which to live and to accomplish their plans. Typically, the young person looks upon illness, disability, and death as rather abstract or remote possibilities if indeed he thinks about them at all. This of course changes markedly as the person gets into middle age.

Middle age bears some resemblance to adolescence in that it too is a period in which significant biologic changes occur in the individual. The male observes that he has less hair on his head and more on his chest; the torso may become more rounded, especially the lower abdomen, and the legs may become thinner and less strong; various health problems, some minor and others more major, often develop; there is usually a perceptible, slow decline in resilience or endurance; while intellectual functions are usually well preserved there may nonetheless be a decrease in the person's inclination to learn new concepts. The menopause occurs signaling to the woman that the child-bearing period of her life has come to a close.

If libidinal drives wane in middle age, or if their waning is anticipated (correctly or not) by the individual, there may be an apparent recrudescence of sexual interest. This may in part arise from a feeling, common among middle-aged persons, that life is passing them by. Thus, it is as if certain gratifications must be achieved "now or never." This is an especially pressing issue if the individual feels cheated by life whether as a result of his or her own constrictedness, or because of a too-early marriage which deprived the person of sufficient experimentation, or for some other reason. The "cheated" person, feeling that his sexual drives or abilities are on the wane or soon will be, may set about to make up for lost time. This is the so-called dangerous age for both sexes and may be accompanied by an adolescentlike striking out from home base, getting involved in affairs, or perhaps divorce and a new marriage. This may be an occasion of profound pathos, a frenetic search for new beginnings, new experiences, and a flowering of pseudoyouthful behavior which may mask underlying despair.

Middle age is also a time when the individual may, in a healthy and constructive way, take stock of himself and his situation. Sometimes this stock-taking results in the appropriate relinquishment of long-held but unrealizable ambitions. This relinquishment, which usually occurs piecemeal, is often accompanied by sadness or depression but it may also result in a less burdened life, one in which the individual is fairly "settled," as though he has hit his stride and is continuing to be productive while released from the strain of burdensome ambitions, and is thus freer to enjoy the fruits of his labor. As this occurs, the individual often begins to devote a somewhat larger share of his or her time and energy to the welfare of the community at large, including the needs of the older and younger generations.

Relinquishment arising from a different source may also occur in middle life. For example, the giving up of old roles and satisfactions and the search for new ones may be necessitated by the departure of the youngest child for college, career, or marriage, or by other environmental circumstances which disrupt or terminate important roles and relationships. It is most frequently in this period of life that the individual experiences the deaths of his parents and it is not rare for a sibling or a peer to become seriously ill or to die. These experiences, in combination with the biologic changes taking place in the person, help to reduce or abolish the youthful illusion of indestructibility. The middle-aged person experiences time very differently than do younger persons: time seems to pass ever more quickly and the person becomes increasingly aware of the essential transience of the human condition. With this change in his Weltanschaung, the middle-aged person often develops a more peaceful and keen appreciation of experiences in the "here and now." All of these and other changes of middle life may result in a reordering of priorities, a casting aside of false idols, and a focusing on the things "that really matter" in life: in a word, integrity and wisdom.

Eventually, the diminishments of old age result in a narrowing of functions, varying degrees of disability, and, in conjunction with a decreasing circle of friends and family from sickness and death, there ensues a progressive restriction of activities and increased dependence on surviving relatives and institutions. In some ways, of course, the increased dependence upon others for life support in old age can be looked upon, as it classically has been, as a "second childhood." But the comparison of old age with childhood is quite superficial. The elderly person, dependent though he may be, is often called upon to make adjustments to new and bewildering situations and to deal somehow with the inevitable multiple losses that impinge upon him, including the near-term prospect of final separation from all he has ever known. It is little wonder that regressive behavior and depression are so commonly seen from middle age to the end of the life span. As with the adolescent, a most vital factor in helping the elderly person to live out his life with a sense of wholeness and dignity is that of continuing to recognize him as a person who still counts, who is loved, and who is useful and needed.

SOME CHARACTERISTICS OF PSYCHOLOGIC HEALTH AND MATURITY

It seems fitting to close this chapter with a brief description of some of the characteristics which are associated with the attainment of health and maturity. This is not the same as attempting to describe a particular personality type or profile because the several features mentioned below are present in people who are otherwise not alike at all.

The psychologically healthy and mature individual, while interested and responsive to others, has a relatively stable, inwardly derived feeling of self-esteem. He is able realistically to appraise his own abilities and limitations and has developed life goals in accordance with them. In the pursuit of these goals he is able to foresake the immediate gratification of desires when this is necessary.

It is a mark of maturity to be able to place trust in others to a degree that is appropriate to the current situation and to past experiences with the persons involved. The mature person is able to form lasting, important relationships in which he feels empathy and love.

In general, the coping responses of the mature person are based upon accurate assessment of present reality in the light of relevant past experi-

21

ences and are therefore much less rigidly stereotyped or repetitive than are those of immature and neurotic individuals. This is not to say, however, that the mature person does not exhibit patterns of behavior which reflect his own particular attitudes, values, goals, and habitual modes of coping.

The psychologically healthy person is not, of course, free of problems. When he experiences a failure, as he inevitably will, he is disappointed but not devastated. No one is totally conflict-free and everyone has moments of feeling anxious or frightened and thus has developed his or her own repertoire of defenses. Similarly the healthy person may have minor fluctuations in mood for no apparent reason but these are generally brief and not incapacitating.

REFERENCES

1. Aitken-Swan J, Paterson R: The cancer patient. Delay in seeking advice. Br Med J 1:623, 1955
2. Brenner C: An Elementary Textbook of Psychoanalysis. New York, International Univ Press, 1973
3. Erikson E: Childhood and Society. New York, Norton, 1963
4. Freud A: The Ego and the Mechanisms of Defense. New York, International Univ Press, 1946
5. Hamburg D, Adams J: A perspective on coping behavior. Arch Gen Psychiat 17:277, 1967
6. Mahler MS: On human symbiosis and the vicissitudes of individuation. J Am Psychoanal Assoc 15:740, 1967
7. Paterson R: Why do cancer patients delay? Can Med Assoc J 73:931, 1955

PART
II

PSYCHOLOGIC ASPECTS OF PHYSICAL ILLNESS

Chapter

3

Perception and Meanings
of Physical Illness

Perception of Initial Symptoms
Meanings of Illness
  Physical Implications of Illness
  Psychologic Meanings
  Socioeconomic Meanings

In the preceding chapter, we discussed some of the ways in which people respond to the stresses of life in general. This chapter deals with psychologic responses to a particular group of stresses in which the physician has a special interest, namely, those associated with physical illness.

PERCEPTION OF INITIAL SYMPTOMS

Usually an individual whose illness begins by producing serious discomfort, functional impairment, or an observable change in his body perceives these changes promptly and begins to weigh their significance, preparatory to doing something about them. However, this is not always

25

the case, especially when the disease process affects higher cerebral function. Some patients with organic brain syndromes seem not to have observed their deteriorating memory, impaired concentration, tendency to get confused, and other signs of declining cognitive functions. It is particularly common for such a patient to be quite unaware of affective blunting and of changes in his customary way of behaving. In the following clinical anecdote, the patient's unawareness of grave functional impairment posed potential hazards for himself and others.

A 60-year-old practicing physician was seen in psychiatric consultation at the requests of his internist and his family. He vaguely complained of "occasional" trouble in finding the word he wanted to say and in understanding other people. In spite of this complaint he nonetheless stated that he had "very little" difficulty in communicating with people and he denied any other serious problem in functioning. On examination, however, the patient exhibited extreme difficulty in expressing himself, being frequently unable to find the right word and tending to misuse words. He was grossly disoriented in time, memory for recent events was very poor, and he became confused when attempting to subtract 7 from 100 serially. The patient was not only unaware of his obviously grave impairment of intellectual functions but also of his striking tendency in recent months to be distant and unresponsive to others, including his immediate family.

It is noteworthy that, in addition to apparent failure to observe the intellectual, affective, and behavioral changes attributable to cerebral damage, the patient with organic brain syndrome may be relatively insensitive to body sensations. For example, moderately obtunded persons are sometimes unaware of the sensation of thirst and thus may tend to become dehydrated unless fluid intake is monitored.

Slowly progressive disease affecting organs of perception may also go unnoticed until the functional deficit is relatively severe: the patient with gradually advancing deafness may go through a period of being annoyed with others for mumbling while remaining unaware of his own difficulty in hearing; bitemporal hemianopsia and other alterations in the visual field including unilateral blindness may go unobserved by the patient for some time and may first come to his attention through the observations of others or when the patient is given a medical examination.

It is possible that the occasional failure of brain-damaged patients to report symptoms of their illness results not from lack of perception of these symptoms but from unconscious denial of them. If that is the case, the denial of illness is a defense against anxiety generated by the perception of symptoms. This sequence of perception-anxiety-denial is also seen in a variety of disorders not involving cerebral impairment. Denial of illness, conscious or unconscious, is always related to what the illness means to the patient.

MEANINGS OF ILLNESS

To understand fully the meanings of illness for any individual patient is a potentially complicated undertaking, for it would entail knowledge of a number of interacting factors: the nature of the illness, the patient's past experience with illnesses in himself and others, the life-setting in which the illness occurs, and the patient's personality which is in part the product of the sum of all his past experiences. In spite of this complexity it is feasible to gain an approximate notion of the patient's feelings and ideas about his illness by listening to his spontaneous comments, his response to questions, and by observing his behavior.[5]

In some respects, the patient's approach to his illness is not unlike that of the physician, differing from the latter's primarily by virtue of the patient's lack of technical knowledge and by the relatively greater influence of his emotional reaction to what is happening to him. The patient's first response to the initial symptom of illness is to decide whether the symptom is important (deserves further consideration) or trivial (can be dismissed).

The hypochondriac patient, being exquisitely attuned to even minor variations in physical feelings and invariably inclined to place ominous interpretations on them, errs in the direction of considering every symptom important. Through his consistent overreaction to minor complaints, he runs the risk of lulling his family and the physician into being insensitive to symptoms which are indicative of organic disease. Less common is the patient who inappropriately interprets physical symptoms as "just psychologic" as was exemplified by the intern described in the first chapter. Often, the patient's apparent dismissal of initial symptoms as insignificant masks an underlying anxiety about them.

Having made the decision that their symptoms are not trivial, most patients (perhaps all) engage in some sort of speculation about the diagnosis and prognosis although usually the patient does not choose to reveal his speculations to the physician. When asked to do so, he may give the famous reply: "You're the doctor—you tell me!" This reponse often stems in part from a fear of looking foolish if he reveals his own tentative "diagnosis" and in part from deeper anxiety about his condition. This kind of resistance can be lessened by assuring the patient that the physician respects his views and wants to be sure that the patient's questions and concerns are dealt with as the examination proceeds.

If the patient has interpreted his initial symptoms as being indicative of some disease of which he is frightened or about which he feels hopeless, or otherwise severely threatened, he may temporarily deny their significance or even their existence. This reaction was shown by the patient described in the preceding chapter who tried to ignore the nodule in her breast and did not seek medical attention until her husband insisted upon it. The ways in which an illness can be perceived as threatening to the patient are numerous; for descriptive purposes it is convenient to place them in three categories: physical, psychologic, and socioeconomic. In real life these three categories are closely interrelated and in all of them illness can be perceived as threatening the patient with loss of one kind or another.

PHYSICAL IMPLICATIONS OF ILLNESS

The patient's interpretation of the physical meaning of his symptoms is basically determined in the same way in which he interprets any other event in his life: presently perceived data are interpreted in the light of related past experiences and this interpretation is influenced by conscious and unconscious fantasies and emotions. For example, the patient with severe headache is especially apt to think of brain tumor if he had a relative who died of a brain tumor; this will be a particularly frightening thought if the patient had a guilt-ridden, ambivalent relationship with the deceased relative.

Undoubtedly, the most basic fear associated with any serious illness, especially one which requires hospitalization and/or surgery under general anesthesia, is that of death. Also common are fears of other kinds of loss: loss of a limb or other body part, loss of an important function, loss of body image through disfigurement, and loss of a sense of well-being.[1,3] The patient's apprehensions may or may not be realistic: for example, the person facing transurethral prostatectomy may incorrectly assume that the operation will inevitably render him sexually impotent unless this is specifically discussed with him.

PSYCHOLOGIC MEANINGS[4-6]

Any serious illness can be perceived by the patient as threatening him with an undesirable or even unbearable change in his image of himself as a person, ie, his self-image. For example, the alteration of the physical image of the self (body image) following myocardial infarction is often followed by feelings of apprehension and sadness which are eventually overcome as the patient learns to live within the limitations imposed by his illness; that is, the alteration in body image occasioned by the illness leads to changes in self-image to which the patient must adapt. For some patients the threat of physical illness to feelings of self-worth is extreme. This is, of course, apt to be the case if the illness (or its treatment) is perceived by the patient as gravely interfering with patterns of behavior essential to the maintenance of self-esteem or to the avoidance of anxiety. Thus the individual who cannot stand the thought of being passive, dependent, and nonproductive and who therefore has always been very active, competitive, independent, and successful, may conceive of an illness such as myocardial infarction as being nothing short of catastrophic. This is illustrated by the following case report.[2]

Mr. A. was a 45-year-old married man and father of several children. Until the onset of the present illness, he had been in good physical health. His illness began with an episode of chest pain accompanied by weakness, restlessness, and sweating. Upon the urging of his associates, he reluctantly consulted the family physician. Following the examination the physician informed him that he was having a "heart attack," and advised him to enter the hospital and that complete bed rest for a period of time would be necessary. The patient rejected the diagnosis, stated that the chest pain was already much better, and refused any further examination or treatment. The next day, at work, the pain returned and the patient called his physician again. The latter, upon repeating his advice to the patient and again encountering sharp resistance, suggested that a consultant be called. When the consulting internist confirmed the diagnosis of myocardial infarction, the patient angrily denounced him too as incompetent and again returned to work. He got along fairly well for three or four days until he experienced another attack of severe chest pain, went into shock, and was taken by ambulance to the nearest hospital.

At the hospital, the patient continued to deny that there was anything wrong with his heart. When another cardiologist unequivocally confirmed the previous diagnosis, the patient intellectually accepted it and agreed to remain in the hospital. However, he ignored the modified coronary regimen that was carefully explained to him, got up at will from his bed, puttered around his room at various small tasks, and, via the telephone, kept in close touch with the small factory of which he was president. In brief, although he now verbally accepted the fact of his illness, his nonverbal behavior reflected continuing denial of it as well as stubborn defiance of the medical team.

The patient talked surprisingly freely to the psychiatric consultant. From early in life, he had striven to be the best at everything he had undertaken. For him, sports and games had never been opportunities for relaxation and fun; rather, they represented competitive challenges and his participation in them was loaded with tension. He had approached his business in the same way and, for many years, it had been a consuming grind. He had little ability to delegate responsibility to others and had attempted to run the factory singlehandedly. He was determined to be extremely successful with no help from anyone.

One could speculate about the "underlying problems" reflected in this man's character structure and overt behavior. It is reasonable to hypothesize that he had a great deal of anxiety about persisting infantile, passive-dependent longings. One might wonder if he had an unconscious image of himself as being small and weak, like a child posing as an adult. In any event, it was apparent that he had never truly resolved his inner problems, but had dealt with them through a combination of repression, denial, and reaction formations. The latter were crucial in warding off intense anxiety and feelings of helplessness and worthlessness, ie, he had to be constantly active, self-assertive, and extremely independent, striving for and achieving success whether in business or on the golf course. Therefore, when he was afflicted with an illness that threatened to deprive him of crucial character defenses, he responded by massive resistance.

About two weeks after admission the patient developed unremitting chest pain, made worse by physical activity. He appeared ashen and weak. At this time he no longer actively opposed the therapeutic regimen and remained at bed rest. With acceptance of the inescapable fact that he was gravely ill, he became despondent and stated that he could not accept the possibility of partial recovery. He made it clear that if he could not get "completely well" and return to his life-long pattern of hyperactivity, unfettered by a heart condition, then he hoped that he would die. A few days later he did.

In the above patient the intense conflict between the illness (or, more accurately, the patient's conception of the illness) and crucial character defenses evoked the following sequence: stubborn denial, defiant behavior, worsening of the illness, breakdown of denial, submission to the illness, followed by despondency and a wish to die. We may note that this patient exhibited, in extreme form, personality features that have been described as frequently present in coronary-prone individuals. Conflict between illness or treatment and psychologically important defenses is not uncommonly seen in one form or another.

Even in the absence of severe conflict, patients may grieve because of actual losses necessitated by illness such as separation from family and friends, relinquishment of cherished plans or goals, loss of a favorite activity or type of recreation, loss of ability to sire or bear children, and so on.

The patient may consciously interpret illness as a punishment for past sins or there may be more vague feelings of guilt, stemming from largely unconscious sources. In either event, the patient may derive a certain amount of satisfaction if he feels that his suffering has expiated him from guilt. Often, however, the guilt-ridden patient who sees his illness as punishment fears that the fates have even more suffering in store for him. Such a person may have a prior history of constantly fearing that something bad is going to happen to him and reacts to physical illness as if the long-dreaded doomsday had arrived.

Not everyone, of course, sees illness as pure adversity. Mention has already been made of the guilt-ridden person whose illness is expiatory. Illness can also be welcomed if it enables an individual to escape from a difficult life situation or if it offers him a "respectable" way of satisfying his needs to rest and be cared for. The longer an illness lasts the more it is apt to become incorporated in the patient's defenses and psychologic needs. The person who welcomes illness and finds it gratifying has no difficulty in shifting into the "sick role" but is apt to have trouble in giving it up during convalescence.

SOCIOECONOMIC MEANINGS

The possible social and economic effects of incapacitating illness are innumerable and, in some instances, may confront the patient with distressingly conflictful choices. The mother of small children, for example, may feel apprehensive and guilty about leaving them to enter the hospital, especially if her husband cannot afford to take time off from work to be with them or if he seems indifferent. Tactful inquiry into the patient's life situation and the consequences of illness and treatment, especially hospitalization, should always be made. The medical social worker can be helpful in assessing the social and economic impact of the illness and in assisting the physician to manage this aspect of the patient's care. The well-trained social worker is aware of resources in the community, such as the availability and costs of homemaking services, with which many physicians are relatively unfamiliar.

Direct discussion with key members of the family is essential in the discernment and management of practical problems raised by the patient's illness. The fact that the physician shows an interest in the patient's life situation, especially in relation to the complications introduced by illness, while at the same time being respectful of the patient's and family's sensitivity and need for privacy, is in itself reassuring to the patient. Many patients hesitate to tell their physician of their worries concerning the family or work because they feel the physician may regard this as not part of his job.

Occasionally, of course, illness is seen by the patient as an economic opportunity, leading to the procurement of disability income or litigation for damages, real or imagined, which are thought to have produced the illness. In the latter instance, if it is likely that a substantial part of the patient's illness or disability has a nonorganic basis, a lump-sum settlement for damages would seem preferable to periodic payments that are contingent upon continuing disability.

The patient's perception of symptoms and the meanings of illness are important determinants of his attitudes toward the therapeutic regimen and of his feelings and behavior if hospitalization is required. These aspects of illness behavior are discussed in the following two chapters.

REFERENCES

1. Bandry FD, Wiener A: The surgical patient. In Strain JJ, Grossman S (eds): Psychological Care of the Medically Ill: A Primer in Liaison Psychiatry. New York, Appleton, 1975, chap 10
2. Imboden JB: Psychosocial determinants of recovery. In Lipowski ZJ (ed): Advances in Psychosomatic Medicine, Vol. 8. Psychosocial Aspects of Physical Illness. New York, Karger, 1972, p 142

3. Kiely WF: Coping with severe illness. In Lipowski ZJ (ed): Advances in Psychosomatic Medicine, Vol. 8. Psychosocial Aspects of Physical Illness. New York, Karger, 1972, p 105
4. King SH: Perceptions of Illness and Medical Practice. New York, Russell Sage Foundation, 1962
5. Lipowski ZJ: Psychosocial aspects of disease. Ann Intern Med 71:1197, 1969
6. Strain JJ, Grossman S: Psychological reactions to medical illness and hospitalization. In Strain JJ, Grossman S (eds): Psychological Care of the Medically Ill: A Primer in Liaison Psychiatry. New York, Appleton, 1975, Chap 3

Chapter

4

Patient Noncompliance with Medical Treatment: Contributory Factors and Management

Patient's Psychologic Status
Social and Family Circumstances
Characteristics of the Illness
Characteristics of the Therapeutic Regimen
Patient – Physician Relationship

From the foregoing discussion of the perception of initial symptoms and the meanings of illness, it is apparent that at times the patient may decide not to seek medical help when he should, or he may decide to seek medical help but do so with much ambivalence. The frequency of ambivalence about treatment, whether present from the beginning of treatment or developing later, is evidenced by the fact that a very large number of patients who go to the physician for help fail to comply with the treatment regimen he prescribes. In spite of the fact that noncompliance obviously constitutes a common and important complication in management, most physicians have a low index of suspicion for it.

The factors contributing to compliance or noncomplicance can be grouped according to their relations to (1) the psychologic status of the patient, (2) social and family circumstances, (3) characteristics of the illness, (4) the therapeutic regimen, and (5) the patient–physician relationship. These factors and their management implications are discussed below.[1-4]

PATIENT'S PSYCHOLOGIC STATUS

In order for the patient to seek treatment and to comply with the therapeutic regimen it is essential that he be (1) sufficiently uncomfortable or concerned about his illness to do something about it, (2) hopeful that effective help is possible, (3) confident in the physician or physicians to whom he has access, (4) unaverted from following through with the treatment plan by the development of strongly negative feelings and attitudes, and (5) thoroughly knowledgeable about his role in the implementation of the treatment plan.

It is not rare for a patient to underestimate grossly the potential importance of his complaints (and therefore the diagnostic evaluation and treatment) because of a lack of factual information. An attitude of inappropriate casualness or obvious indifference alerts the physician to this possibility which can be confirmed or ruled out by tactfully asking the patient appropriate questions to discern his ideas about his condition. *In engaging the patient in an educational dialogue the physician aims to fill in important gaps in information, correct distortions, and promote the formation of a working partnership with him.* In doing this, the physician takes care to avoid engendering unnecessary anxiety or anxiety that is so severe that the patient is frightened away.

Not uncommonly, a blasé attitude or an exaggerated air of indifference, which may herald noncompliant behavior, masks underlying fear. The covertly fearful, potentially noncompliant patient may also appear superficially cold or tend to be hostile, caustic, skeptical, and critical. Here too it is possible for the underlying anxiety to be related to serious factual misconceptions regarding the symptoms, illness, or treatment, in which case the management approach remains essentially an educational one.

An occasional patient may observe his own symptoms and be sufficiently concerned about them to seek medical help while at the same time engaging in *partial denial* of their import. Partial denial is not necessarily maladaptive since it may serve temporarily to cushion the impact of the illness, help the patient to hold himself together while he attends to important personal affairs, and, in general, give him time to muster his resources. For example, the patient, on being informed of some serious or ominous finding, may temporarily seem paradoxically casual or even cheerful, while at the same time appropriately making arrangements for entering the hospital and doing whatever else his physician has advised.

In this instance, the physician may be certain that the inappropriate cheerfulness does not reflect lack of information but is part of the patient's adaptation to current stress. As long as the partial denial is not accompanied by behavior which interferes with evaluation and management, the physician is well advised to leave well enough alone.

When, however, denial of illness does result in behavior which jeopardizes the patient's participation in treatment, as was the case in the myocardial infarction patient described in Chapter 3, the physician must attempt to ascertain the factors promoting the denial and develop a management approach. In practice, these two processes of evaluation of patient behavior and management are virtually inextricable and must be tailored to the needs of the individual patient.

One or more of the following are sometimes useful in the management of noncompliance arising from partial denial of illness.

1. Engage the part of the patient's ego which does accept the fact of his illness. By this it is meant that the physician supportively reminds the patient that to some extent he obviously recognizes his need for medical attention as evidenced by the fact that he kept his appointment to see the physician or entered the hospital or had the prescription filled and so forth. This acknowledgment is followed by matter-of-factly pointing out that other aspects of the patient's behavior, however, seem to contradict his realistic acceptance of the illness. This comment can then lead into a nonjudgmental inquiry into the patient's feelings, attitudes, and fantasies relating to the illness and treatment.
2. Attempt to allay or reduce underlying anxiety. The most effective way to reduce anxiety is to help the patient bring into the open his concerns and fears such as may arise from some dire interpretation of a particular symptom, a conviction that he will be left an invalid, or a feeling that his illness is something to be ashamed of or that his condition is hopeless. Even if the underlying problem is not completely resolved, and it seldom is, the sharing of it with the physician can be extremely helpful and may enable the patient to face the current stress and to comply with the plan of treatment. The temporary administration of a minor tranquilizer such as chlordiazepoxide or diazepam may be a useful adjunct to this approach.
3. At times, when medically permissible, it may be necessary to postpone or modify the management plan if some aspect of it poses a particular problem. It may be helpful, for example, to delay hospitalization for a day or two if this is likely to promote the patient's acceptance and cooperation. The patient might learn more of what to expect in the hospital by making a visit and talking with some of the nursing staff. Another source of anxiety-relieving information is another patient who has already dealt with the condition; for instance, colostomy clubs can

provide invaluable support to patients contemplating this major surgery.

4. Psychiatric consultation may be indicated but should only be instituted after the physician has initiated exploratory discussion of personal feelings and problems with the patient and feels that the consultation is necessary to help understand and alleviate the noncompliant behavior. The physician should fully discuss with the patient the reasons for psychiatric consultation and must be careful to avoid the impression that the patient is being rejected, ie, that the physician wants someone else to pay attention to the patient's personal problems because he himself is not interested in them.

In addition to lack of accurate information and denial-producing anxiety, there are other aspects of the patient's psychologic status which may promote noncompliant behavior. Prominent among these are lack of trust in physicians and others, an attitude of rebellion against authority figures and restrictive therapeutic regimens, difficulty in accepting a relatively dependent role, and perception of the treatment plan as an intolerable frustration of important psychologic needs. These will be discussed further later in this chapter and in the following chapter in which various psychologic reactions during hospitalization and their management are described.

Occasionally, noncompliance with the therapeutic regimen is associated with depression. In these instances, the noncompliant, depressed patient may feel guilty and thus feel that he does not deserve or want to get well. If his depression has gone unrecognized, the patient may also feel that the treatment plan prescribed for him is not directed at his main difficulty. The key to management rests upon recognition of the depression and the institution of appropriate treatment for it by the physician or by referring the patient to a psychiatrist.

SOCIAL AND FAMILY CIRCUMSTANCES

The physician should always pay careful attention to the patient's family situation and socioeconomic background. Lack of money or transportation and preoccupation with pressing family or occupational demands may gravely interfere with the patient's ability and willingness to comply with the management plan. In this situation it is sometimes tempting for the physician himself to ignore these aspects and to rationalize this posture by saying that his job is to prescribe treatment, the patient's to carry it out. However, tactful but frank discussion of the home and job situation may well lead to the discovery of practical aids to facilitate participation in treatment. A skilled social worker is often invaluable in the assessment of these problems and in the utilization of community resources in their solution.

CHARACTERISTICS OF THE ILLNESS

It is likely that when the illness produces considerable discomfort such as pain, shortness of breath, or weakness which is substantially improved by the prescribed drug and which recurs when the medicine is not taken, the patient will comply with treatment. However, if the illness or problem is relatively "silent," such as uncomplicated essential hypertension or hypercholesterolemia, the likelihood of noncompliance is enhanced. In these instances, noncompliance should be anticipated and counteracted by a clear explanation of the benefits of treatment and by follow-up visits in which compliance is reinforced by informing the patient of the results of ongoing treatment.

CHARACTERISTICS OF THE THERAPEUTIC REGIMEN

Treatment plans most likely to evoke noncompliant behavior are those which are complex, require substantial changes in the patient's daily habits, and in which the benefits are imperceptible to the patient or are slow to appear. When the therapeutic regimen has one or more of these features the physician should anticipate possible noncompliance and encourage the patient to express his feelings about the treatment and to ask questions about any aspects of it. Not only are complicated treatment plans more apt to cause the patient inconvenience, but they are also harder to understand. It is always necessary to describe the treatment in comprehensible terms and, through tactful discussion, ascertain that the patient in fact does comprehend the treatment plan. If it is medically sound to simplify the treatment and to reduce its interference with the patient's daily routine, this should be done. For example, single daily administration of a drug is more apt to be complied with than three or four divided doses. If it is anticipated that the administration of a drug should be continued for some time after symptomatic remission has been achieved, it is important to discuss this with the patient for many people "forget" the medicine as soon as they are feeling better.

Sometimes the therapeutic regimen does not merely create inconvenience in the patient's daily life but actually conflicts with important psychologic needs. For example, adhering to a low-calorie diet is made doubly difficult if the overweight patient is in the habit of seeking relief from depressive feelings through eating. In such a case, treatment of the depression should accompany or take precedence over a strictly dietary approach to the patient's problem with excessive weight.

The adolescent patient with diabetes may find a restrictive therapeutic regimen particularly onerous because it conflicts with his age-appropriate need to be "like" his peers and with his struggle for autonomy. The physician may avert or minimize behavior management problems with the diabetic adolescent if he lets him know that he is aware that the patient may have troubling feelings about his illness and its treatment, that at times he may be unhappy or angry. This interest in the adolescent's feelings must be genuine, ongoing, and manifest to the patient but must not be smothering or intrusive. It is an inviting but not coercive interest and is accompanied by a willingness to consult with the patient about various practical aspects of the treatment plan and to respect his observations and suggestions.

Strict bed rest or instructions to "slow down" may seem impossible to the person whose feeling of worth has been almost entirely derived from being active and competitive. This situation may pose exceedingly difficult dilemmas for both patient and doctor and may make it necessary to "negotiate" a compromise treatment plan which, while it falls short of the ideal, has a better chance of being carried out.

PATIENT–PHYSICIAN RELATIONSHIP

In the last analysis, the quality of the patient–physician relationship is probably the most crucial variable in determining compliance with treatment plans. In the daily work of the busy practitioner, failure to take the time for truly adequate communication is perhaps the most common and damaging deficiency of modern medicine. If the physician is to maximize his effectiveness, he must cultivate a relationship of mutual respect, offer explanations in a clear manner, invite questions and expressions of feelings and ideas, and be alert to evidence of psychologic and other obstacles that stand in the way of full patient cooperation. *A relationship in which trust and rapport are established enhances the likelihood that the patient will be able to talk about his misgivings and tensions rather than express these feelings through noncompliant behavior.* Tactful exploration of the patient's values, habits, life style, and relationships with other people, including past experiences with other physicians, provides important clues to the probability of noncompliant behavior and to the tailoring of treatment plans to the individual patient.

REFERENCES

1. Blackwell B: Patient compliance. N Engl J Med 289:249, 1973
2. Gillum RF, Barsky AJ: Diagnosis and management of patient noncompliance. JAMA 228:1563, 1974
3. Gross HS: A practical approach to non-compliance in primary care. Md State Med J 24:55, 1975
4. Rosenstock IM: Patients' compliance with health regimens. JAMA 234:402, 1975

Chapter

5

Psychologic Reactions During Hospitalization: Their Evaluation and Management

Some General Features of Hospitalization
Separation
Reunion
Uncertainty
Transference
Regression
Special Clinical Situations
Intensive Care Areas
    ILLNESS - RELATED FACTORS
    ENVIRONMENTAL FACTORS
Hemodialysis for Chronic Renal Failure
Surgery
Psychologic Disturbances
Anxiety
Depression
Acute Brain Syndrome
Psychosis without Apparent Organic Basis
Miscellaneous Behavior Problems
    UNCOOPERATIVE BEHAVIOR
    SELF-DESTRUCTIVE BEHAVIOR
    COMPLAINING AND DEMANDING BEHAVIOR
    SEXUALLY PROVOCATIVE BEHAVIOR

Management
  Patient–Physician Relationship
    CONFIDENCE AND RAPPORT
    TAILORING APPROACH TO PATIENT'S PERSONALITY
  Physician's Response to Denial
  Conceptual Clarification
  Anticipating the Patient's Experiences
  Confrontation
  Modification of the Management Plan
  Environmental Modification
  Medication
  Psychiatric Consultation

In the instance of serious illness that requires hospitalization, the prospective patient must not only recognize his need for medical help and seek it, he must also temporarily relinquish his customary social role upon entering the hospital, adapt to the complexities and uncertainties of life in a modern hospital, and, during convalescence, relinquish the sick role and return to his preillness position in society to the extent that recovery allows. Usually this whole process, though always accompanied by emotional reactions of various sorts and degrees, proceeds without a serious hitch. Sometimes, however, emotional reactions and behavior patterns do develop which threaten seriously to compromise treatment and impede recovery; these reactions constitute genuine complications of the illness or treatment and require thoughtful evaluation and management.

SOME GENERAL FEATURES OF HOSPITALIZATION

The hospitalized patient is confronted with the prospect of placing himself almost totally in the care of people who, with the possible exception of his personal physician, are apt to be complete strangers. In the hospital he loses control over many aspects of his daily life: other people or hospital routine determine when he wakes up in the morning, when and what he eats, when and how many people may visit him, whether he stays in bed or not; physical examinations, laboratory procedures, x-rays are scheduled for him, sometimes without his knowledge; medicines are "ordered." He is apt to have much less privacy than he is accustomed to; nurses, nurses' aides, students, interns, residents, technicians, and his attending physician may pop into his room at all hours of the day (and evening) with or without a warning knock.

He is subjected to a number of procedures which have a "leveling" effect: certain personal belongings are removed for safe-keeping; he is tagged with a wristband, clothed in a short gown more or less open in the back; he endures repeated history-taking and physical examination by assorted persons (especially in a teaching hospital), has various body orifices inspected and probed, is carted here and there by wheelchair or stretcher; and in general he is in a relatively passive position of having things done to him which he often does not understand by people who frequently are in a hurry and who may seem to him to be more concerned with other patients who are more ill than he.[13]

SEPARATION

Hospitalization usually separates the patient to a considerable degree from the important people in his life and from customary sources of satisfaction in recreation and work. Socially and vocationally, the hospitalized person is temporarily "out of the running" for in a sense he must step aside while life goes on. While some patients welcome this aspect of the experience, perceiving it as a needed respite, many others feel saddened, grieved, or fearful that the presumably temporary separations caused by hospitalization may turn out to be permanent. The latter threat may arise from consciously entertained possibilities of death or invalidism or it may be connected with a fear of being replaced, eg, by an ambitious, younger person who is pinch-hitting for the patient at his place of employment.

REUNION

As with illness itself, hospitalization may afford the patient considerable psychologic gratification.[21] The fact of being seriously ill allows the patient an opportunity for socially approved passivity and dependence. In addition, members of the family may "gather around" and, in various ways, show their love and concern for the patient. Sometimes old rifts between the patient and relatives or friends are closed, at least temporarily, and the patient's illness brings about a kind of family reunion. Perhaps these psychologically "positive" aspects of illness and hospitalization contribute to an interesting phenomenon that psychiatrists have often observed, namely, the sometimes striking remission shown by schizophrenic patients who become physically ill. Temporary improvement may also be seen in other types of emotional disorder when physical illness intervenes.

A 65-year-old widower had suffered for many years with a severe obsessive-compulsive neurosis. A great deal of his waking life was taken up with innumerable, complicated obsessions and rituals. In the course of time, he had become estranged from his two children, partly because they found his constant worrying and ritualistic behavior difficult to tolerate. As the patient's estrangement from his children progressed, he became more and more concerned that certain thoughts (obsessions) which came into his mind would cause something terrible to happen to them. He really knew that this could not be so, that one person's thoughts could not harm another person. But the anxiety was there nonetheless and the patient was compelled to engage in lengthy prayers and other rituals to protect his loved ones from harm.

When the patient developed an acute intestinal obstruction, requiring emergency surgery, his children became very concerned. Their relationship with the patient changed. Instead of being icy, hostile, and distant they manifested much warmth, visited him frequently throughout his hospital stay, and kept closely informed about his condition. Throughout the period of hospitalization, the patient was impressively less beset with obsessions and compulsions than he had been for many years. Following hospitalization, many of the old obsessive-compulsive symptoms returned, as did the estrangement from his children, though not to the degree that existed prior to the surgical illness.

UNCERTAINTY

There is always some degree of uncertainty in the patient's mind regarding the danger to life and limb, duration of hospital stay, the likelihood of pain and other suffering, and the ultimate outcome of his hospital experience. While it is true that it is beyond the power of the physician totally to remove the patient's uncertainty (for this would be tantamount to removing reality), it is within his power to engage the patient in matter-of-fact discussions about his experiences and concerns; this is done, not with the aim of completely alleviating anxiety or a harmless defense against anxiety such as the noninterfering use of denial, but for the purpose of correcting distortions and supplying the patient with information which realistically enhances feelings of security and hope.

During the course of hospitalization, especially if occasioned by prolonged, severely incapacitating, or life-threatening illness, the patient almost invariably undergoes some degree of regression and develops a relationship with the physician which is heavily colored by transference.

TRANSFERENCE

Transference is the displacement of feelings and attitudes from important relationships in earlier life to someone in the present. The rapid development of intense transference in the hospitalized patient's relationship with physicians and nurses is fostered by several factors.

1. In terms of the degree to which the patient is utterly dependent upon others, the experience of hospitalization more closely resembles that of infancy or childhood than does almost any other situation of adult life. As a result, old feelings, expectations, and attitudes, deriving from the dependency situation of early life, are mobilized and manifested in overt or disguised form in the patient's relationships with those currently caring for him. That is, the patient is now "in the hands" of the physician and nurse as he had once literally and figuratively been in those of his parents. Old issues of trust or distrust, of being cooperative or rebellious ("doing what he is told," being a good boy or good patient), of perceiving those in whose charge he now is as loving, caring, reliable, and competent or the reverse are to some extent reexperienced.

2. As already noted, the chances are that many or all of the staff are strangers to the patient and even his attending physician may be relatively unknown to him. This relative anonymity of the physicians and nurses facilitates the patient's imparting to them attributes derived from earlier experiences with authority figures, especially his parents. The patient is also apt to draw upon his prior experiences with other physicians and nurses in making assumptions about those with whom he is currently dealing.

The two preceding sets of factors combine to promote intense transference: being in a position of extreme dependence upon the physicians and nurses for his comfort and for his very survival, the patient almost invariably has some measure of anxiety. This anxiety is allayed considerably by the development of a strongly positive transference in which the patient imputes to the physician (and others who are perceived as critically important to his welfare) the omniscient and omnipotent qualities which his parents seemed to possess when he was a small child. In other words, the hospitalized person's situation is such that he needs to feel that his physician is the best and is totally committed to his welfare. In this connection, physicians have repeatedly noted that often the patient regards what the physician says as virtually infallible, even though the patient may actually know very little about the physician. This faith in the physician may have a very powerful therapeutic influence. It is possible, for example, that some of the early success with internal mammary artery implantations was a result of the patient's faith in the surgeon rather than myocardial revascularization.[24] Positive transference, even when it entails rather obvious overvaluation of the physician, does not ordinarily pose a problem, is psychologically useful to the patient, and the physician does well simply to accept it.

44

There may, however, be transference reactions of a negative nature. Warning clues to this type of transference are obtained when the patient, in relating his history, reveals a pattern of being critical of other physicians who have cared for him in the past. It may not be possible to prevent the development of negative transference. If the patient becomes resentful, distrustful, and critical it is important to assess the possibly realistic justification for his feelings. If such an assessment, which should include not only the physician's own dealings with the patient but other factors including attitudes of other members of the staff, leads one to the conclusion that the patient's negative criticisms are unrealistic or overdone, it is quite possible that one is observing transference distortions. Recognition of this possibility helps the physician to maintain professional objectivity, to be tolerant of the patient's feelings, and to engage him in discussion of them. Usually, however, it is not helpful to attempt to interpret the childhood origins of transference feelings to the patient.

REGRESSION

In the course of prolonged hospitalization and severe illness, many patients revert to forms of behavior, feelings, or modes of thinking which were characteristic of them at a much earlier stage of life. Strictly speaking, intense transference is itself a type of regression. Regression in hospitalized patients may take many forms depending upon its severity and upon defensive reactions to anxiety engendered by the regression.

Regression, in its moderate and more usual form, represents an understandable, useful adaptation to hospitalization. The patient becomes quite centered upon himself, especially upon his physical sensations and symptoms, comes to rely extensively upon others to meet his needs, and accordingly may develop unrealistic expectations of response by the staff to his complaints or requests. He is therefore more upset by minor provocations than normally and, as described above, may derive considerable comfort by exaggerating the competence, dedication (to the patient), and general goodness of his physician and other members of the staff. The patient who comfortably experiences the regressed, dependent state often becomes irritable during the recovery phase when he is called upon to relinquish the legitimized gratifications afforded by the illness.

Not all patients experience regression comfortably. The patient may feel quite threatened by his own dependency needs, or may lack a sense of basic trust in those who care for him and may therefore need to assert his autonomy. For these and other reasons, a variety of complicating behavior patterns may emerge in the course of hospitalization. These will be discussed later in this chapter.

SPECIAL CLINICAL SITUATIONS

INTENSIVE CARE AREAS

In response to the needs of critically ill patients and to the advantages of concentrating advanced equipment and specially trained personnel in defined areas within the hospital, intensive care units (ICU) and coronary care units (CCU) have been widely developed. These intensive care areas have proven their usefulness in critical care medicine. It has become recognized, however, that the incidence of serious psychologic disturbance among patients in these units is relatively high and, further, that the emotional stress experienced by the staff, especially nurses, is greater than that in other parts of the hospital.

Although the term "ICU syndromes" has been used to refer to the mental or emotional disturbances observed in intensive care patients, it does not appear that there is a qualitatively unique syndrome that characterizes these disturbances. In intensive care areas, as elsewhere in the hospital, patients may develop anxiety, depression, delirium, and paranoid states, and may present a wide variety of behavioral problems which require management. The relatively high incidence of psychologic disturbances in these areas is apparently due to a number of factors as described by McKegney,[20] Kornfeld,[15] Cassem and Hackett,[5] and others.[10]

Illness-related Factors   Patients are not admitted to intensive care areas, of course, unless they are very seriously, usually critically, ill. If cardiac arrest, respiratory cessation, or shock has occurred at any point in the course of illness, the resulting cerebral anoxia may affect cognitive functions and behavior, depending upon its severity and duration. Numerous other physiologic consequences of illness such as hyponatremia, hyperkalemia, hypoglycemia, and uremia may profoundly alter higher cerebral function.

With the growing population of older persons, it is to be expected that a substantial number of patients in intensive care areas are elderly and have some degree of cerebral impairment due to senile and arteriosclerotic processes. These patients are predisposed to an acute brain syndrome superimposed on their chronic conditions. The use of barbiturates in elderly patients may be associated with increased confusion and agitation.

A minority of patients admitted to intensive care units have self-inflicted wounds or have taken drug overdoses. The emotional or behavioral conditions which led to the suicidal attempt become part of the clinical picture when the patient regains consciousness.

The psychologic meaning of the acute illness to the individual patient is of extreme importance in determining emotional and behavioral reactions, as was evidenced by the patient with myocardial infarction described in Chapter 3. In describing their extensive experience with psychiatric consultations on a coronary care unit, Cassem and Hackett noted that anxiety reactions tend to occur most frequently on days 1 and 2 in the CCU, depression on days 3 and 4, and that behavior management problems had a bimodal distribution, peaking on days 2 and 4.[5] These authors have accordingly described a "natural history of the emotional reactions" of normal persons to myocardial infarction. Upon admission to the CCU, having just experienced life-threatening, crushing chest pain, the average person feels considerable anxiety. With symptomatic improvement, particularly if evidence of cardiac damage is equivocal, denial is mobilized and the patient may protest hospitalization and insist upon returning to work (the first peak of "management behavior problems"). By the third or fourth day, the average patient with a confirmed diagnosis of myocardial infarction becomes more aware of the implications of his condition and despondency often occurs. At this point, some patients with conflicts centering on dependency and passivity begin to display irritating, provocative behavior.

Environmental Factors   The physical design and atmosphere of intensive care areas vary considerably from one hospital to the next and increasingly have received thoughtful attention as the importance of environmental stresses on patients and staff has become apparent. Nonetheless, in many intensive care areas, the patient is surrounded by a physical setting which may seem strange and frightening to him. The patient is apt to be deprived of normally present, orienting sensory cues such as clocks, newspapers, windows, and a regular schedule of meals. On the other hand, he is overloaded with sensory stimuli which may be quite anxiety-provoking such as the visual and auditory signals of monitoring equipment, the occurrence of crises which summon physicians and nurses to a nearby bed or room, deaths of fellow patients, and the general tension that sometimes pervades the atmosphere of an intensive care unit. The patient may be almost immobilized by tubings of various sorts and wires connecting him to equipment. The overhead light may remain on, physicians and nurses are at his side frequently to perform necessary chores, and he hears the moans and groans of other patients. In this environment, the patient may be seriously deprived of sleep for several days or more. The combination of sensory monotony, sensory overload, and sleep deprivation further predisposes the patient to the development of emotional disturbances and confusion.

It should also be noted that the availability of sophisticated monitoring equipment, vital though it is, can result in the substitution of telemetry for personal contact between staff and patient; this is particularly apt to occur when the unit is unusually busy or understaffed.

HEMODIALYSIS FOR CHRONIC RENAL FAILURE[4,7,8,14]

Although patients who receive ongoing dialysis for chronic renal disease are usually managed only partially or intermittently in the hospital, it is convenient to consider some of the psychologic aspects of this form of treatment in this chapter. The stresses undergone by these patients usually are severe and stem in part from the effects of the underlying renal insufficiency and in part from the treatment regimen. The latter requires the patient to conform to rather strict dietary restrictions and to two or three times weekly dialysis sessions which are time-consuming, inescapable, and sometimes alarming to the patient (especially the novice) who is aware that a portion of his blood is out of his body and in the machine during the procedure. This whole situation forces the patient not only to modify his daily life in conformity with treatment requirements but also to be dependent upon the personnel of the dialysis unit or, in the event of home dialysis, his wife or other helper.[26]

The ability to tolerate the restrictions, changes in life routines, and dependence on the machine and people varies a great deal from one person to the next. Some persons repeatedly deviate from the treatment program in ways which are deleterious or life-threatening, others conform but become excessively "dialysis-centered," and still others seem to do what is necessary and continue actively to pursue their goals and interests which may be modified to suit their current situations.

Most patients requiring dialysis are uremic to some degree at one or more times in the course of their illness, and during uremic episodes higher cerebral function is frequently impaired sufficiently to produce an acute (reversible) brain syndrome or delirium. This condition may at times be mild enough that it is only detectable by doing a mental status examination. Impairment of orientation, memory, and other cognitive functions prevents the patient from resuming certain kinds of activities if he is discharged from the hospital and may also interfere with his grasping and retaining instructions given to him about the dialysis procedure, diet, and other aspects of management.

The patients often feel tired and weak, and are confronted with a basically unending, incurable disorder though they may live in hope of receiving a kidney transplant or of future technical improvements in the dialysis procedure. Kidney transplantation itself is loaded with grave uncertainties and the hope for a kidney to become available may even be tinged with guilt if it entails the accidental death of the future donor. In the meantime, the dialysis patient may be caught in a situation of not being clearly well or clearly sick. He is, as Landsman has pointed out, a "marginal man."[16]

Somewhat surprisingly, in view of the severe stresses impinging upon these patients, the incidence of overt, psychotic disturbances does not appear to be high. Not surprisingly, many patients, especially those whose occupations have required much physical activity, find it very difficult to find a productive, satisfying role for themselves. Some patients become depressed. Wise has pointed out, however, that there is a "pitfall" to be avoided in diagnosing depression in patients with chronic renal failure, ie, apparent depression may be correlated with the presence of uremia and may lift as the uremia is alleviated by treatment.[27]

SURGERY [9,17,22,29]

Patients who undergo surgery and require postoperative care in a recovery room for a substantial period of time are, of course, exposed to the psychologic stresses already described for all ICU patients. In addition, there are special aspects of the surgical patients' experience which merit attention. These include the particular features of the illness or conditions for which surgery is required and of the operation itself.

If the illness has been of long duration and has been utilized for the avoidance of anxiety or for other psychologic gain, there may be considerable difficulty in rehabilitation following successful surgery. Through the development of new symptoms or the continuation of old ones, a substantial degree of invalidism may persist in spite of good physiologic results from surgery. This was observed, for example, by Kaplan[12] in his study of patients who underwent mitral commissurotomy and by Eifrig et al in patients following pericardectomy.[6] On the other hand, those patients who have a history of continuing difficulty in adapting to or accepting the incapacitation of illness may quickly reestablish preillness patterns of living after successful surgical intervention.

It is not rare for patients with deep-seated emotional problems to develop somatic complaints and actively to seek a surgical operation. While there may be transient symptomatic relief, the underlying problems remain unaltered and new symptom formation usually occurs. Thus it is not rare for the patient with long-standing or recurrent conversion hysteria to have a history of polysurgery.

Occasionally the performance of surgery to correct a psychogenic symptom may precipitate emotional decompensation. This may be particularly apt to occur when the patient's psychologic problem is expressed in one major physical symptom such as preoccupation with an objectively minimal cosmetic deformity of the nose (especially in males) or impotence.

While it is reasonable to assume that there is always some degree of anxiety prior to surgery, there does not appear to be clear evidence of a

49

positive correlation between degree of overt preoperative anxiety and emotional disturbance in the postoperative period. It may well be, however, that denial of anxiety preoperatively is associated with a greater likelihood of subsequent psychologic disturbance. In addition, patients who believe they will die during or following the operation may carry a higher risk of fatality than do patients who believe they will survive. In the former instance, surgery should be delayed, if possible, and psychiatric consultation obtained.

The surgical procedure itself may have actual or symbolic consequences which pose considerable stress for the patient. Loss of a limb, mastectomy, colostomy, orchidectomy, and hysterectomy are among surgical procedures which may result in the patient's feeling functionally diminished, unworthy, incomplete, or unlovable as a man or woman.[18] In such patients it is not rare for depression to occur days, weeks, or months after the operation.

Postoperative psychosis with evidence of acute organic brain syndrome is not rare. Its incidence is increased by any procedure which enhances the likelihood of compromised cerebral function such as prolonged anesthesia, cardiac bypass in open-heart surgery, and the use of barbiturates, especially in the elderly. The presence of chronic brain syndrome, commonly present in older patients, enhances the likelihood of postoperative delirium. Not rarely, a patient with undiagnosed alcohol or barbiturate addiction develops an unexpected withdrawal syndrome following surgery.

PSYCHOLOGIC DISTURBANCES

Effective management of patients who develop psychologic disturbances in the course of hospitalization rests upon accurate diagnosis, including the discernment of significant etiologic factors. As Albert and Kornfeld have pointed out in their study of patients who threatened to sign out of the hospital against medical advice, early diagnosis and prompt intervention may serve to prevent the development of serious behavioral disturbances.[1] Early detection is thwarted by breakdowns in communication between the staff and the patient and between members of the staff.

The variety of psychologic disturbances observed in hospitalized patients is considerable and depends in part upon the patient's personality or characteristic modes of coping with stress as well as upon the nature of the particular stresses to which he is currently subjected. The following is a brief review of some of the more commonly observed psychologic difficulties experienced by medical and surgical patients.

ANXIETY

The anxious patient may be restless, tend to glance frequently around the room or toward others as if he is hyperalert, have sweaty palms and tremor, look worried or apprehensive, and have difficulty in relaxing and falling asleep. He may at times appear tensely rigid. The specific content of fears and apprehension may be revealed in spontaneous remarks by the patient or in response to tactful inquiry of a sort which conveys a certain empathy by the questioner.

DEPRESSION

Sad or expressionless facies, slowness of motor behavior and speech, apathy or apparent lack of interest, anorexia, difficulty in falling asleep, fitful sleeping, and early awakening all point to the presence of depression. The patient may or may not verbally express feelings of depression or sadness, pessimism, hopelessness or despair, and worthlessness. Some depressed patients may keep such feelings to themselves for fear of alienating physicians and nurses, especially if they are perceived as being concerned only with the physical aspects of the patient's illness. Not uncommonly, symptoms of anxiety and depression occur together.

ACUTE BRAIN SYNDROME

Reversible impairment of cognitive (including perceptual) functions, often accompanied by varying degrees of excitement and fear, may occur in a wide variety of medical and surgical illnesses. Disorientation and memory impairment are often not discernible on casual observation and may only be detected by doing a mental status examination. The timing of the examination is important since delirium is often characterized by marked waxing and waning, exacerbations frequently occurring in the evening. Frightening illusions and hallucinations involving visual, auditory, and tactile modalities and paranoid delusions which are poorly systematized and changeable may occur.

PSYCHOSIS WITHOUT APPARENT ORGANIC BASIS

In predisposed individuals grave psychologic decompensation may occur even in the absence of physical impairment of higher cerebral function. Hypomanic states manifested by hyperactivity, hypertalkativeness, and euphoria or irritability are occasionally seen. Paranoid states, manifested by extreme distrust and delusions of being watched, poisoned, or conspired against may sometimes develop. These severe states of psychologic decompensation may result from conflict between defensive behavior patterns and the immobilization or enforced dependency imposed by the treatment situation. Less commonly they are precipitated by the inadvertent compromising of crucial defenses through symptom removal.

MISCELLANEOUS BEHAVIOR PROBLEMS

There are a number of behavior management problems which defy traditional classification and which may be associated with all of the psychologic disturbances described above.

Uncooperative Behavior   Intense anxiety, with or without organic cerebral impairment, can evoke defensive denial of illness and therefore of the need for treatment. Grave suspiciousness, delusional mistrust, understandable misinterpretation of environmental cues, and confusion may lead to anger and fear which are manifested by refusal to cooperate with the staff or by threats to sign out against medical advice. More rarely, the depressed patient may be uncooperative because he feels his condition is hopeless or that he is unworthy of treatment. *The associated emotional disturbance is usually manifest before the eruption of blatantly uncooperative behavior or threats to sign out.*

Self-destructive Behavior   Behavior with potentially injurious or lethal consequences is frequently seen in delirium. Impaired judgment, relatively poor impulse control, and panic may lead the delirious patient to pull out intravenous tubing, strike at the nurse or aide, wander from his room, or jump out a window. Planned, deliberate suicide attempts, on the other hand, are usually associated with depression.

Complaining and Demanding Behavior   The patient who complains of symptoms which are out of proportion to the organic illness or which have no organic basic at all quickly becomes regarded as a "crock." Excessive symptomatic complaints may or may not be associated with other complaints related to the diet, service, room temperature, staff attitudes, or some other feature of the hospital. Generalized complaining is usually associated with demandingness, the patient asking the staff at all hours of the day or night to give him something he needs or to correct some allegedly intolerable deficiency.

Complaining, demanding behavior often arises from covert anxiety in that it reflects the patient's insecurity and his need constantly to reassure himself that someone is available and responsive to his needs. This type of behavior may also arise from the patient's need to exert control over his environment and thereby to recapture a measure of the autonomy which was his prior to hospitalization. Complaining and demanding behavior may be an expression of thinly veiled anger, distrust, and a desire to manipulate staff members.

Ironically, the behavior usually has a "positive feedback" effect in that it alienates the patient from the staff and thus may result in a degree of actual neglect which then fuels further complaints and demands.

Sexually Provocative Behavior   The patient whose self-concept, particularly his image of himself as a virile male, has been threatened by real or imagined consequences of the illness may attempt to bolster self-esteem by engaging in a variety of sexual overtures directed toward the nurses and female physicians. This behavior may take the form of jokes, making passes at the nurse, and exhibitionism.

MANAGEMENT[2,3,9,11,19,22,23,25]

PATIENT–PHYSICIAN RELATIONSHIP

Confidence and Rapport   Of basic importance in general medical management and in minimizing the likelihood of severe emotional disturbance is the establishment of a physician–patient relationship in which confidence, trust, and open communication are fostered. Experienced physicians and nurses often convey the all-important fact of their technical competence through an unaffected professional manner of unruffled, sometimes casual self-assurance in their dealings with the patient. Each experienced clinician has his own unique way of establishing rapport with the patient and knows the value of informing him in clear, understandable language of diagnostic and treatment plans and progress.

Tailoring Approach to Patient's Personality[2,3]   It is clear, however, that the way the physician relates to the patient is not only influenced by the physician's own personality but also by the personality and current emotional needs of each individual patient. Bibring and Kahana[3] have pointed out the usefulness of tailoring one's approach according to the salient characteristics of the patient's personality and the value of utilizing one's knowledge of important psychologic needs in influencing the patient's behavior. For example, the suspicious, paranoid person responds best to an approach of firmness, accuracy, and careful avoidance of ambiguities. The schizoid person can be expected to be somewhat aloof and distant; the physician, while encouraging him to ask questions or to clear up any matter about which he may be doubtful or worried, nevertheless respects the schizoid patient's need for privacy. The obsessive–compulsive person tends to reduce anxiety by learning all the facts and attaining intellectual mastery of situations; the physician can help such a patient to meet these needs by judicious review of clinical procedures and of the various relevant aspects of the hospital environment. On the other hand, the excitable, histrionic, or hysteric patient, while certainly needing to be informed of the essential facts of his clinical situation, may be in greater need of an opportunity to ventilate his feelings, fears, and fantasies. The patient who has always taken pride in being strong, self-sufficient, and in control can be tactfully reminded that he plays an active role in the treatment process and that in going through hospitalization and treatment he is doing his part to get back on his feet; the physician further supports this type of patient by eliciting his opinion about various issues relating to the clinical situation and utilizing those suggestions which have validity.

PHYSICIAN'S RESPONSE TO DENIAL

As noted elsewhere, denial may be a useful coping response which gains the patient time to muster his resources and tides him over a particularly frightening phase of the illness experience. An example of this is the person who, while complying with the treatment regimen, displays an affect of cheerfulness, as if the full impact of his illness has not yet sunk in. In this situation, the physician does well simply to refrain from challenging the denial. He judiciously supports the patient's morale but is careful to avoid being unrealistically optimistic.

Denial that leads to overt disavowal of the fact of illness or which is manifested by behavior that implies disavowal can pose extremely difficult management problems for which there are no simple solutions. In these instances psychiatric consultation is often indicated.

The psychologic approach to the patient who presents a behavior problem stemming from denial of illness and of need for treatment includes tactfully calling to the patient's attention the fact that part of him must recognize his need for medical attention as evidenced by the fact that he did, after all, consult the physician, entered the hospital, and, depending upon the individual patient, has partially complied with treatment requirements. This represents an attempt to support the reality-testing part of the patient's ego and to nurture a sense of alliance between patient and physician. Depending upon the patient's response, the physician then attempts to help the patient deal with the fears or other feelings which have given rise to the denial. This may need to be done in graded steps and a logical place to begin is simply to ask the patient to talk about any troubling feelings or worries that may be bothering him, even if they do not seem to be connected with his illness. Psychiatrists have long observed that persons who talk about their feelings and fantasies with someone they trust are less likely to act upon them than are people who keep everything to themselves. The goal then is to foster the patient's verbalization of his ideas, fears, or worries and, when appropriate, to correct distorted concepts of the illness or treatment. Conceptual clarification of significant aspects of the patient's condition and treatment is an important part of management even when the patient is not engaged in treatment-interfering denial.

CONCEPTUAL CLARIFICATION

It is wise never to assume that the patient has an accurate grasp of his illness and treatment and their implications. Some explanation to the patient of his condition and of what he can expect as treatment progresses is in order prior to or at the beginning of hospitalization. The completeness and detail of such an explanation are tailored to the situation and needs of the individual patient and should be followed by inviting the patient to inform the physician of any questions or concerns which arise. The variety of disturbing conceptual distortions which may arise in the course of serious illness is enormous. Some patients may secretly assume that cancer is never curable, that persons with heart attacks can never work again or engage in sexual intercourse, that prostatectomy always causes impotence, that the heart is weaker during sleep and therefore sleeping is dangerous, or that the low-voiced corridor conversations of rounding physicians carry some ominous implication. Sometimes the physician can anticipate distortions but more often he must learn of their existence from the patient; this requires a continuing attitude of interest in what the patient is experiencing.

ANTICIPATING THE PATIENT'S EXPERIENCES

It may strengthen the patient's ability to adapt to the various phases of the illness if he is given some forewarning as to what he is likely to experience. For example, the patient who has been told that he will have some pain in the postoperative period and that he will be encouraged by the nurses to cough will know that these experiences are "normal" and that his surgeon, who predicted them, is in control of the situation. If the patient with myocardial infarction is informed that he will likely feel some weakness for a period of time after his discharge from the hospital, he will not be so dismayed by that symptom or so apt to interpret the weakness as evidence that his heart is weaker than either he or his physician had thought.[28]

CONFRONTATION

When the patient has been engaging in disturbing or provocative behavior it may be useful for the physician or nurse to confront him with what he is doing. The confrontation should be simple, direct, matter-of-fact, and should not be done in anger. The confrontation may be accompanied by some discussion of the possible reasons for and consequences of the disturbing behavior. For example, after pointing out his behavior to the complaining-demanding patient, the physician may comment that many patients need to assure themselves that the staff is on the job but that calling them for trivial reasons is apt to be self-defeating. When confrontation is necessary it is important to give the patient an opportunity to express his side of the problem, and occasionally it is helpful to clarify or modify the management plan.

MODIFICATION OF THE MANAGEMENT PLAN

To continue with the complaining-demanding patient, the physician will find it helpful to discuss the behavior problem with the nurses and other members of the staff who have the most contact with the patient. Staff resentment should be aired and resolved, which may not be too difficult if the nurses are aware of the physician's interest and that he has discussed the problems with the patient. It may be useful, particularly when the demandingness is primarily serving to allay anxiety, for the physicians and nurses to make a point of making frequent, brief visits to the patient's room on a more or less regular schedule. The resulting display of interest and concern even when the patient has not called may remove the need to be demanding.

The patient who finds strict bed rest intolerable or who is threatened by passivity and dependence on others and is therefore trying to restore his sense of autonomy may be irritable, stubbornly negativistic, or resistant and generally difficult. It is often bolstering to the self-esteem of such a patient for the physician to discuss selected aspects of management with him and to elicit his ideas and suggestions. Working out a compromise therapeutic regimen with the patient may not only result in reducing the onerous aspects of treatment but may also give the patient a needed feeling of partial control or at least active collaboration with the physician.

ENVIRONMENTAL MODIFICATION

The environmental stresses described for intensive care areas often exist to some degree in other parts of the hospital as well. Careful attention to the patient's environment is important in the prevention and management of adverse psychologic reactions. All patients, particularly those who are delirious or are likely candidates for development of delirium, should be provided with individually appropriate, orienting, sensory cues such as a daily newspaper, a view of a window to differentiate day from night, frequent contacts with staff, and clear communication. If possible the patient should have a reasonable degree of privacy and should not be bombarded by disturbing stimuli such as the signals of his own monitoring equipment; the moans, groans, crises, and deaths of other patients; having an overhead light constantly on; and so forth. Careful attention should be paid to providing an environment in which the patient can get to sleep and, if possible, not be repeatedly awakened. If the patient is confused or suicidal, a responsible person should remain with the patient at all times.

MEDICATION

The overtly anxious, hospitalized patient often requires a minor tranquilizer such as diazepam (Valium), 5 mg to 10 mg bid or tid, and a mild sedative in the evening. It is useful to explain to the patient that he will be given the medicine for a few days and that its purpose is to help him to feel less tense and more relaxed. Barbiturates should be used with caution since their use is sometimes associated with paradoxial excitement and increased confusion, especially in the elderly patient.

Antidepressant drugs may be indicated in depression and one of the major tranquilizers in psychotic states. The management of toxic psychoses secondary to withdrawal in cases of alcohol and sedative addiction requires administration of an appropriate substitute medication at adequate dosage with carefully graduated reduction over a period of days (see Chaps. 9 and 10).

PSYCHIATRIC CONSULTATION

Psychiatric consultation is indicated in severe behavioral or emotional disturbances particularly when psychosis, marked anxiety, or depression is suspected or if the patient's behavior is seriously jeopardizing, directly or indirectly, the patient's safety and recovery. The utilization of the psychiatric consultant for disturbances of lesser severity depends on whether the primary physician feels the need for assistance in the development of a plan of management. Not rarely the emotionally troubled patient himself requests the consultation.

In any event, when the physician decides to request psychiatric consultation his first step is to discuss the need and potential usefulness of the consultation with the patient. The patient's receptiveness to the consultation, and hence its value, are enhanced if the patient understands at least some aspects of the problems for which the psychiatrist will see him. The psychiatrist himself will be more effective if he is thoroughly briefed by the referring physician as to the medical background and problems of the patient than if he sees the patient blind. Some patients may feel rejected and that their primary physicians are abandoning them to the psychiatrist. This can be averted by making it clear that the psychiatrist will function as a consultant to the primary physician who will continue to be responsible for the patient's care.

REFERENCES

1. Albert HD, Kornfeld DS: The threat to sign out against medical advice. Ann Intern Med 79:888, 1973
2. Bibring GL: Psychiatry and medical practice in a general hospital. N Engl J Med 254:366, 1956
3. Bibring GL, Kahana RJ: Lectures in Medical Psychology. New York, International Univ Press, 1968
4. Brown TM, Ferris A, Parke RC, Paulus DA: Living with long-term home dialysis. Ann Intern Med 81:165, 1974
5. Cassem NH, Hackett TP: Psychiatric consultation in a coronary care unit. Ann Intern Med 75:9, 1971
6. Eifrig DC, Imboden JB, McKusick VA, Canter A: Constrictive pericarditis. Psychologic aspects of convalescence following pericardectomy. J Chronic Dis 13:52, 1961
7. Foster GF, Cohn GL, McKegney FP: Psychologic factors and individual survival on chronic renal hemodialysis. A two year follow-up. I. Psychosom Med 35:64, 1973
8. Greenberg RP, Davis G, Massey R: The psychological evaluation of patients for a kidney transplant and hemodialysis program. Am J Psychiatry 130:274, 1973
9. Hackett TP, Weisman AD: Psychiatric management of operative syndromes. I. Psychosom Med 22:267, 1960
10. Hay DH, Oken D: The psychological stresses of intensive care unit nursing. Psychosom Med 34:109, 1972
11. Hellerstein HK, Friedman EH: Sexual activity and the postcoronary patient. Arch Intern Med 125:987, 1970
12. Kaplan SM: Psychological aspects of cardiac disease. A study of patients experiencing mitral commisurotomy. Psychosom Med 18:221, 1956

13. King SH: Perceptions of Illness and Medical Practice. New York, Russell Sage Foundation, 1962
14. Kolodner LJ: Experiences of a surgeon on dialysis. Md State Med J 22:35, 1973
15. Kornfeld DS: Psychiatric problems of an intensive care unit. Med Clin North Am 55:1353, 1971
16. Landsman MK: The patient with chronic renal failure. A marginal man. Ann Intern Med 82:268, 1975
17. Lane OL, Jr, Ydolfsy SC: Postoperative psychosis in cardiotomy patients. N Engl J Med 284:518, 1971
18. Lindemann E: Observations on psychiatric sequelae to surgical operations in women. Am J Psychiatry 98:132, 1941
19. Lipowski ZJ: Review of consultation psychiatry and psychosomatic medicine. II. Clinical aspects. Psychosom Med 29:201, 1967
20. McKegney FP: The intensive care syndrome. Conn Med 30:633, 1966
21. Mechanic D: Response factors in illness. The study of illness behavior. Soc Psychiat 1:11, 1966
22. Meyer E, Jacobson WE, Edgerton MT, Canter A: Motivational patterns in patients seeking elective plastic surgery. I. Women who seek rhinoplasty. Psychosom Med 22:193, 1960
23. Meyer E, Mendelson M: Psychiatric consultations with patients on medical and surgical wards. Patterns and processes. Psychiatry 24:197, 1961
24. Ross RS: Surgery for coronary artery disease placed in perspective. Bull NY Acad Med 48:1163, 1972
25. Stein EH, Murdaugh J, MacLeod JA: Brief psychotherapy of psychiatric reactions to physical illness. Am J Psychiatry 125:1040, 1969
26. Streitzer J, Finkelstein F, Feigenbaum H, Kitsen J, Cohn GO: The spouse's role in home hemodialysis. Arch Gen Psychiat 33:55, 1976
27. Wise TJ: The pitfalls of diagnosing depression in chronic renal disease. Psychosomatics 14:83, 1974
28. Wishnie HA, Hackett TA, Cassem NH: Psychological hazards of convalescence following myocardial infarction. JAMA 215:1292, 1971
29. Ziegler FJ, Rodgers DA, Kriegsman SA: Effect of vasectomy on psychological functioning. Psychosom Med 28:50, 1966

Chapter

6

The Dying Patient
and His Family

In recent years the care of the dying patient and his family has received a great deal of attention in professional and lay circles. This has occurred largely because of remarkable advances in medical technology.

With the development of sophisticated life-support systems, cardiopulmonary resuscitation, chemotherapeutic intervention in heretofore life-shortening incidental infections, and advances in the various modes of treating cancer, the length of time between initial diagnosis of fatal illness and death has increased significantly. It is therefore inevitable that physicians, patients, and their families have become increasingly concerned with learning how to help fatally ill and terminally ill patients. When looked at superficially this interest may seem to be in conflict with the role of the physician as one whose duty it is to combat death. This conflict of course is more apparent than real for in addition to his obligation to attempt to *cure* the patient of illness and thus to prevent death, the physician has always been presumed to be realistic in his expectations of therapeutic efficacy and to be concerned with the total *care* of the patient, including the alleviation of pain and the facilitation of comfort and peace.

Death and dying have a profound impact on physicians and nurses as well as patients and families. It is not rare in fact for the reactions of the staff to be of kinds that interfere seriously with caring for the dying patient or even interfere with developing a plan for the patient's care. In the following section, we will discuss some physician reactions that may interfere with management. Subsequently, we will describe the overall goals of management of the dying patient, the stages of dying, and the period of bereavement that occurs in those close to the patient after the patient's death.

PHYSICIAN REACTIONS TO DEATH AND DYING

In order effectively to care for the dying patient, it is necessary to think about him, to talk with him, to listen to him, and to maintain a relationship with him until death occurs. For some physicians this is feasible and for others it is extremely difficult. There are many possible factors that can enter into the development of interfering emotional reactions in the physician.[4] As with all human behavior, the physician's response to the dying patient is determined in part by the sum of all the physician's past experiences in life and in part by the particular features of the situation in which he currently finds himself. From his own past experiences and personal development, the physician brings to the dying patient certain concepts, values, and expectations that he has concerning life, death, and himself as a person.

DENIAL OF DEATH

In spite of their experiences with sickness and death, physicians are no more exempt from the tendency to avoid or deny death than are people in general. If in fact one customarily deals with the issue of physical death by not thinking about it and not accepting it as real and inevitable for one's self, then this defense (avoidance, denial) will be sharply challenged each time a dying patient is encountered. When this happens the physician may manifest the continuance of his own denial of death in a variety of behaviors: he may falsely reassure the patient (at a cost of later loss of patient's confidence in him), he may overload the patient with too much information in one sitting in order to get the whole business done with, he may tend to withdraw from the patient, he may unwittingly participate in a "conspiracy of silence" thus contributing to the patient's isolation, or he may simply fail to get across to the patient that he will stand by him to take care of such basic needs as the alleviation of pain and other discomfort.

What should the physician do if he suspects that his own denial of death is powerful and seriously interferes with his effectively relating to the dying patient?

For the short term, he may choose to obtain the participation of someone, perhaps another physician, a nurse, a clergyman, or a social worker, who is comfortable and experienced in working with dying patients. In such an event, the primary physician will usually decide to remain the responsible clinician though delegating part of the management to someone else.

For the longer term, the physician may choose to try to come to grips with the issue of death and of his avoidance of his own thoughts and feelings about his own death. This can be facilitated by having discussions with respected colleagues and friends. The development of an awareness and acceptance of death is not a gloomy, psychologically morbid process. Indeed, persons who achieve this awareness and acceptance report that they become more alive because they become liberated from the superficial expectations imposed upon them by society and are thus freer to pay heed to their own values and goals.

DEATH AS A REBUTTAL OF OMNIPOTENCE

In Chapter 2, we referred to the illusion of omnipotence that is a normal feature during infant and child development. Fantasies of being omnipotent persist to some extent and with varying degrees of conscious awareness into adulthood. As was the case with the human tendency to deny death (which implies a feeling of being indestructible), physicians are by no means exempt from fantasies of omnipotence. Since a basic aim of medical care is to *cure* the patient, the dying patient may symbolize defeat of the physician. To the extent that the physician's own judgment of his professional performance is colored by fantasies of omnipotence, to that extent will he find it difficult to be realistic in his expectations of himself and to accept the inevitability of death without feeling inadequate, guilty, or frustrated. Failure to cope with such feelings by working through the underlying unrealistic expectations of himself can lead the physician to behave defensively when any aspect of the patient's case is discussed or questioned by a colleague or a relative of the patient. The physician also may deal with his own frustration by overtreating the patient, such as by taking extraordinary measures to prolong life in situations where this is inappropriate. It is natural for the dying patient to evoke a reaction of considerable ambivalence in the physician who feels helpless, frustrated, or defeated by the patient's illness. This ambivalence may be expressed in a number of ways, eg, the physician guiltily wishing that the dying patient would go ahead and die.

GENERAL GOALS AND PRINCIPLES OF MANAGEMENT

Stated in its broadest terms, the overall goal of management of the dying patient is essentially no different from that of any other patient. As Weisman has said, the objective is to help the patient to "live as well as possible for as long as possible."[12] Therefore, what Weisman has called an "appropriate death" takes into account the quality of life for the dying patient as well as the length of life.

The following goals are of paramount importance in the management of dying patients. They are not listed in order of importance since the choice of which to consider first will depend upon the individual patient and his needs at any particular moment in the course of his illness.[2,3]

1. Alleviation of physical discomfort. It is important not only to provide current relief from pain or other discomfort to the extent that is practical, but also to instill a feeling of confidence on the patient's part that this aspect of his care will continue to receive consistent, careful attention. In part this message is conveyed nonverbally through the physician's manifest attentiveness and in part by frequent listening to what the patient has to say and tactfully inquiring into his state of comfort.
2. Prevention of unwarranted loneliness and isolation. To a considerable extent dying is an inherently lonely experience. Often, however, it becomes more lonely and isolated than it has to be. This is the case when the patient, for whatever reason, is avoided by physicians, nurses, and relatives. Loneliness and isolation are also enhanced when no one is free to talk with the patient about what is happening to him even though everyone, including the patient, knows that he is dying. The alleviation or prevention (partial) of loneliness and isolation entails

frequent, though often brief, visits with the patient and a willingness to converse with him in accordance with the patient's own level of awareness, interest, and concern at any particular point in time. Sometimes this may mean simply sitting with the patient, perhaps touching his hand, in silence for a few minutes. The physician will also assist the patient's relatives to cope with their own feelings in a way that will facilitate appropriate contacts between themselves and the patient.

3. Taking care of unfinished business. When a relationship characterized by trust and good communication has been established, the patient is in a position to reveal to the physician, nurse, or close relative certain personal matters that he wishes to take care of while there is still time. This may involve financial or business affairs, such as making a will, making sure the family knows where certain papers are kept, and so forth. The "unfinished business" however, may be of a more personal, emotional nature. The patient may need to talk about and work through residual psychologic conflicts that he finds disturbing. He may need to achieve a reconciliation with one or more persons with whom he has had a troubled relationship. The mother (or father) of young children may need to satisfy herself regarding arrangements for their care after she has gone. Finally, the patient may wish to make his farewell to close relatives or friends.

One physician should be in charge of the patient's care and be prepared to carry through from the initial stage of informing the patient and family of the patient's serious illness to telling the family of the patient's death and being of assistance to them during the period of bereavement. Yet, this central physician need not, and probably should not, do all this alone. Other staff, including other physicians, nurses, social workers, and chaplains, can all contribute to the care of dying patients. The primary physician will work with some or all of those members of the staff who have continuing contact with the patient so that their approach to him is a consistent one. By this it is not meant that everyone should behave exactly the same way to the patient, but that each person relates to the patient in his own individual way while taking into consideration the opinions and experiences of other members of the staff.

In the following section, specific issues of management that are associated with the various stages of dying will be discussed.

STAGES OF DYING

Kübler-Ross described the following stages of dying: denial, anger, bargaining, depression, and acceptance. Not every patient will go through all five stages.[7] Some will show evidence of more than one stage at the same time; others may go back to an earlier stage and then progress forward to the achievement of quiet acceptance and peace.

For purposes of discussion, the process of dying, when viewed from its psychologic aspect, will be considered as beginning at the time the physician informs the fatally ill patient (and family) that he has a serious illness. It is not advisable to tell the patient that there is no chance of recovery or that he has only a certain amount of time left. The patient does have a right to know that he has a serious illness, that treatment is available, and that all will be done for him that can be. The patient is thus given a message of grave import but is also given hope at the same time. Some patients will press for a specific diagnosis or for this or that detail regarding treatment and such information can be given to him, but in a way that does not remove hope or hold a fatal outcome to be a certainty. If the patient asks if the illness is necessarily fatal, the physician can reiterate that the illness is a very serious one or even that one cannot be sure of the outcome at this time (which is true).

The physician thus attempts to tell the patient the news accurately and in small pieces, so to speak. He does not overwhelm the patient with a mass of details which the patient probably won't remember anyway, and he is careful to inform the patient of whatever treatment is available. In the first session in which the physician informs the patient he should allow plenty of time so that neither he nor the patient will feel rushed and so there is ample opportunity for questions and answers.

The responsible members of the family should also be told. The physician should give the family accurate information as he did the patient but may choose to provide more details. If the physician suspects that the patient has not yet grasped the seriousness of his situation, he should be sure the immediate family understands. It is usually wise to inform the family in stages also rather than all at once, especially if the initial reaction is that of being shocked or stunned.

Frequently, the patient's reaction after he has been given the news of his illness is that of denial. Thus the patient may go about his business as if he had not been informed of his serious illness or he may show his disbelief by seeking the opinion of other physicians. It is as though the patient has said to himself, "no, not me, it can't be true!" and believed this.

The physician does not attempt to challenge or override the denial which the patient uses in this initial stage or, for that matter, in later stages of the illness unless the denial results in behavior which interferes with important treatment. In that event, the physician carefully reviews with the patient the fact of his illness, the diagnosis, and the advisability of treatment. When this is done, the physician continues to be careful to remain both truthful and hopeful, eg, explaining the probable usefulness of treatment but without indicating that it will result in permanent cure.

Gradually the patient struggles to comprehend the seriousness of his situation and, as time goes by, the message that he will die. During this phase of dying, it is important to be able to listen to the patient and to respond to him truthfully when he asks questions about his condition. The patient himself may tentatively venture the opinion or offer a hint that he is dying and if he does so he should not be contradicted or offered false reassurance.

ANGER

As the truth of his dying dawns upon him the patient commonly reacts with anger. He may say to himself and to others: "Why did this happen to me? Why me!" He resents being singled out, chosen for death, and the seeming unfairness of it all is very difficult to bear. As anger develops, the patient becomes irritable, and demanding, and may take a hostile, reproachful attitude toward everyone with whom he comes into contact. Perhaps he is really angry at fate or God but is taking his anger out on the nearest available targets.

The physician who is aware of this stage of anger so frequently experienced by the dying patient is in a position not to react defensively or with angry rejection of the patient. The physician knows that it is not he or other staff or relatives toward whom the patient is really angry. The physician's understanding of the patient's anger enables him to listen to the patient, to allow the patient to ventilate his feelings, and to assist other staff and relatives to attain a healthy measure of objectivity and tolerance. Patients for whom being in active control of all aspects of their lives has always been important may fear and resent the loss of control over their own destiny that dying brings. When this is the case it may be helpful to enlist the patient in active participation in his own care and in planning for future care to the extent that is feasible.

BARGAINING

The patient may partially resolve his angry feelings and ward off depression for a while by engaging in what Kübler-Ross has called "bargaining." Bargaining entails a degree of denial combined with a magical expectation of cure or of prolongation of life if the patient says or does certain things.

The latter may involve being a good patient by doing everything the physicians and nurses ask of him or it may involve prayers or promises to be fulfilled if granted the time in which to fulfill them. Here too the physician listens to the patient, allows him to bargain, but does not confirm the patient's unrealistic expectations. Eventually the bargaining attempts fail (although medically unpredicted recoveries do occur) and the patient again becomes angry and/or depressed.

DEPRESSION

The patient recognizes the apparent inexorableness of his dying as though he has answered the question of "why me?" with "why not me," though these actual words may not be uttered. Depression comes as people prepare to die. There are several factors usually present which contribute to depression: the failure of bargaining, persistent or recurrent pain or other discomfort, and the multiple disappointments and losses which the process of dying and the prospect of death entail. The dying patient may feel that he has already lost his role as a useful, needed, or attractive person. Unrealized hopes and ambitions leave him feeling unfulfilled. He feels lonely and faces the prospect of giving up all his relationships with those whom he loves. At this stage the continued availability of the physician and others who are willing to listen to the patient when he chooses to discuss his feelings or simply to sit quietly by him when he chooses to be silent is important in counteracting his isolation and in providing him with support. The physician can be extremely helpful to the patient at this stage by alleviating physical discomfort and by seeing if there are any personal affairs with which the patient needs help.

ACCEPTANCE

As the dying patient mourns the profound losses of all which he has and loves he begins to divest himself of emotional attachments, eventually even to those who are dearest to him. In the process of this progressive "letting go," the patient may or may not talk about or review some aspects of his past life. In this phase the patient frequently achieves a quiet and peaceful acceptance of the approaching end. At this stage it is not unusual for the patient to wish to be alone or, if someone is with him, to be silent. Kübler-Ross has commented on the dignity and apparent equanimity of the dying patient who has worked through the depression and mourning of his losses and has achieved acceptance of his state.[6]

The stages listed above are a useful description but it is worth reemphasizing that they are not to be interpreted too literally, especially the notion of one stage following another in orderly progression. Denial in various forms and degrees may repeatedly appear and disappear prior to final acceptance and one may see varying admixtures of denial, anger, bargaining, and depression at more or less the same time.

It must also be noted that the physician may observe developments in patient or family that lead him to request psychiatric consultation. The psychiatrist who has had experience in consultations on medical and surgical services is apt also to have had experience with dying patients and bereaved families. The excessive and interfering use of denial by patient or relatives and the development of suicidal risk are among the problems for which psychiatric consultation may be helpful.

PROLONGATION OF LIFE

There has been much discussion about the extent to which physicians should go in prolonging the life of hopelessly ill patients. We have found the work reported from the Massachusetts General Hospital, Boston, and Beth Israel Hospital, Boston, to be informative and useful in developing an approach to this difficult problem.[1,9,10]

The plan for care of any critically ill patient should include an attempt to assess the probability of his survival as a neurologically intact person. This probability may need to be reassessed daily. If plans for therapy, based on this prediction, include a less than maximum effort to preserve life, the patient and his family must participate in this decision, although they should never be forced to make it themselves, without support of the primary physician. After discussions of the sort described earlier, patient and family will be well enough informed, and acquainted enough with the primary physician, that they can have a vital share in decisions about how, and for how long, to continue therapy aimed at delaying death.

The patient may be able to participate in this decision at the time of his illness or he may have already expressed his choice in the form of a living will. The latter may include a statement such as "If my death is near and cannot be avoided, and if I have lost the ability to interact with others and have no reasonable chance of regaining this ability, or if my suffering is intense and irreversible, I do not want to have my life prolonged. I would wish, rather, to have care which gives comfort and support, which facilitates my interaction with others to the extent that this is possible, and which brings peace."[1]

This statement offers a starting point for the individual choice which the patient and family must make. The principle of this is that the patient and/or family express a preference, and the physician is responsible for judging whether or how best to carry out the preference. Laws are being drafted and passed in various states which may make clearer both the responsibilities and the immunities for the physician attending the dying patient.

THE PLACE OF DYING

Not all patients die in the hospital. Another organized form of care for the dying is provided by the hospice, based upon traditional and religious practices of care for the seriously ill. In England, Dr. Cicely Saunders has founded modern hospices, offering sound medical care for terminal cancer patients. Features include judicious and unstinting use of analgesics, warm attention by trained and emotionally secure staff, and generally unlimited visiting. Patients offer support to each other as well. These specialized hospices are also appearing in this country.[5]

Patients may choose to spend their final days at home, and in many instances this can be a help in allowing the family to participate more and in lessening the isolation of the dying patient. Some families can do this; others, whether at home or in the hospital, need to be supported in refraining from a prolonged bedside vigil which can drain them. Physicians and nurses need to care for the families as they care for the patients.

Especially at home, but in any instance of a patient's dying, the question arises of the family's being at the bedside at death. With patients who have been made comfortable, this seems very possible and indeed desirable. The patient and family can offer support to each other and the family can know personally how things were at the moment of death.

THE BEREAVED FAMILY

Although there is considerable variation among individuals, it is possible to make some generalizations about the process of grief. Among the important variables that influence the reactions of those who have lost a loved one is the length of time between first learning of the serious or fatal nature of illness and the death of the loved one. When the dying has been a relatively slow process, the spouse or other close relative is apt to go through various emotional stages (which may or may not be coordinated with those of the dying patient) similar to those of the dying patient. When dying has occurred slowly and has been accompanied by considerable physical discomfort and progressive emaciation, the bereaved relative may understandably accept the death of the patient as not only inevitable and natural but also as a welcome release. In such instances, grief has begun prior to actual death although even here the utter finality of death is not usually completely comprehended until the event has occurred.

When dying has been rapid, or death has occurred suddenly, or when the relative has not been able to get past the stage of denial during the patient's dying, little or no anticipatory grief has occurred and therefore the grief process takes place mainly or entirely after the death of the patient.

Parkes has described three stages of grief: numbness, yearning and protest, and disorganization.[8] Parkes' conclusions are based in part on a study of 22 London widows under age 65 who were periodically interviewed during the 13 months following the death of their husbands. As one would expect, there is much in common between Parkes' stages of grief and Kübler-Ross' stages of dying although they are not identical. In contrast with Parkes' study, one gets the impression that much of Kübler-Ross' experiences with the family concerned the period prior to death. It is useful for the family physician to supplement his own personal and professional experiences with the observations made by others in order to develop an appropriate notion of what to expect when a patient or relative has lost a loved one. This knowledge may assist him in understanding and supporting a person who is undergoing grief as well as enabling him more readily to recognize significant deviations from the more usual patterns.

The initial stage of numbness begins after being informed of the death and may last from one day to a week or longer. The person may describe himself as not feeling anything, or feeling as if he were in a dream, or as if he simply could not comprehend the reality, could not let it sink in. Marked tearfulness may occur prior to numbness and may be interspersed during this stage when denial or disbelief momentarily break down and the person is overwhelmed with distress.

The stage of "yearning and protest" is characterized by intense pangs of grief in which the bereaved person pines for the lost one and refusal (often not entirely conscious) to accept completely the fact that the deceased is gone. During this period the person feels sad, tearful, and may have symptoms of anxiety, poor appetite, and insomnia. There may be feelings of anger directed at the deceased person for having left or at the physicians for not having saved the loved one's life. The bereaved person may blame himself for not having done more. Parkes has described the bereaved person in this period as "searching" for the deceased. This may take the form of mentally visualizing the deceased, focusing attention upon his possessions, visiting the grave, mistaking someone on the street for him, or thinking one has felt his presence or heard his voice. Such experiences, including illusions and hallucinations, during this stage are not indicative of impending psychosis. The bereaved person may begin unconsciously to imitate or adopt traits or even symptoms of the deceased, which represents a psychologic attempt to keep the lost one by making him part of one's self.

In most persons, the second stage of grief reaches its peak about two months after the death and subsequently begins to subside. However, many months and sometimes even years after the loss there may occur waves of sadness and pining, often precipitated by some fresh reminder such as a birthday, holiday, anniversary of the death, hearing a certain melody, or visiting a formerly favorite vacation spot.

The third phase of grief, "disorganization," becomes evident as yearning and protest diminish and is characterized by apathy, aimlessness, and disinclination to look to the future or to establish goals and plans. This stage is apt to be less evident and prolonged if the widow's or widower's situation is one in which there are clear expectations and responsibilities such as taking care of the children or earning a living.

There is no clear or readily perceived end-point to the process of grief. Parkes states that two-thirds of the widows he studied were still in the stage of disorganization at the end of their first year of bereavement. Although we know that people never completely get over grieving in the sense of forgetting about their loss, they do eventually renew their interests in social activities and work and make emotional investments in one or more new interpersonal relationships. To do this, to heal the hurt and empty feelings, to find new ways of living without a spouse or parent or child, many people may need assistance.

This can come from several sources. Friends and neighbors offer considerable support in most communities. During the first days of bereavement, in the numb stage, the person needs simple and direct assistance, someone to help him arrange for the funeral and associated activities. Later, in the stage of yearning, when the pangs of grieving come, the person needs unintrusive companionship, in which the person's need for support and for periods of privacy are understood.

Still later, the bereaved person will need to find ways of resuming accustomed patterns and perhaps of starting new endeavors. Neighbors, family, and friends can be important here in providing encouragement. In recent times a movement has developed in which widows work together in self-help groups. On the principle that a person who has successfully coped with a crisis can provide both comfort and guidance to another in the same kind of crisis, these groups have made sizable contributions to many widows' recovery and reentry into active life.[11]

The family physician is in a good position to know when people may need some outside help in dealing with their grief, since he knows the customary habits and patterns of health of his patients. He can offer some direct assistance, support, or advice, or can remind people of other resources and agencies that may help.

He may also detect early signs of complicated or atypical grieving. When a patient shows either no signs of grieving, or exaggerated features such as excessive or prolonged social isolation, unmoderated guilt or anger, or panic attacks, the physician should consider the possibility that the patient is developing a depression which warrants treatment by the family physician or a psychiatrist (see Chap. 14).

REFERENCES

1. Bok S: Personal directions for care at the end of life. N Engl J Med 295:367, 1976
2. Cassem NH, Stewart RS: Management and care of the dying patient. Int J Psychiat Med 6:293, 1976
3. Dunphy JE: Annual discourse. On caring for the patient with cancer. N Engl J Med 295:313, 1976
4. Hinton J: Dying. Baltimore, Penguin, 1972
5. Holden C: Hospices. For the dying, relief from pain and fear. Science 193:389, 1976
6. Kübler-Ross E: Death, the Final Stage of Growth. Englewood Cliffs, NJ, Prentice-Hall, 1975
7. Kübler-Ross E: On Death and Dying. New York, Macmillan, 1969
8. Parkes CM: The first year of bereavement. Psychiatry 33:444, 1971
9. Pontoppidian H, Clinical Care Committee of the Massachusetts General Hospital: Optimum care for hopelessly ill patients. N Engl J Med 295:362, 1976
10. Rabkin MT, Gillerman G, Rice NR: Orders not to resuscitate. N Engl J Med 295:364, 1976
11. Schoenberg B, Gerber I, Wiener A, et al (eds): Bereavement, Its Psychosocial Aspects. New York, Columbia Univ Press, 1975
12. Weisman AD: On Dying and Denying. New York, Behavioral Publ, 1972

PART

III

PSYCHIATRIC PROBLEMS AND DISORDERS ENCOUNTERED IN MEDICAL PRACTICE

Suicidal Behavior and Other Psychiatric Emergencies

Psychiatric emergency refers to any mental or emotional disorder that requires prompt intervention. It is likely that the great majority of psychiatric emergencies that occur outside psychiatric hospitals are first seen by nonpsychiatrist-physicians in their private offices and in the emergency rooms and inpatient services of general hospitals. It is therefore essential for the physician to be able to ascertain that a psychiatric emergency exists, to proceed with diagnostic evaluation to the degree necessary to develop at least an initial plan of management, and to implement the management plan while awaiting psychiatric consultation. As is true with any medical consultation, it is also the primary physician's responsibility to evaluate the opinions and suggestions of the psychiatric consultant and to decide if and when to transfer the primary care of the patient to the psychiatrist.

Psychiatric emergencies are characterized by one or both of the following: (1) behavior which is alarming to the patient or others, and (2) severe subjective distress.

(1) There are many varieties of alarming behavior. One of the most common is that posed by the patient who has made a suicide attempt or who is judged to be in danger of doing so. Any kind of behavior which appears to threaten the well-being or vital interests of the patient or others may be acutely alarming to the patient's relatives or to the patient himself. In addition, behavior or symptoms which are interpreted as indicative of serious illness may be quite alarming even though there is little or no danger to the patient's life. For example, an acute, dramatic conversion reaction, such as sudden paralysis of the legs, is often quite frightening to the patient's family and therefore may require immediate attention.

(2) The two major categories of acute, subjective psychic distress which may constitute emergencies are panic and severe depression.

For purposes of further discussion, it is convenient to consider the problems of suicidal behavior separately and to lump together other forms of alarming behavior arbitrarily under the rubric of "acute behavioral disturbances." The emergency situation sometimes posed by severe depression will be included in the section dealing with suicide. The emergency evaluation and management of panic will be discussed separately.

SUICIDAL BEHAVIOR

Few occurrences in life evoke a more intense welter of emotions in relatives and physicians than does suicide. In fact, the physician, as a person dedicated to the alleviation of suffering and the preservation of life, often must come to grips with the intense ambivalence aroused in himself by a suicide attempt if he is to approach the patient with the same compassion and objectivity that he exercises in other medical emergencies.

DEFINITIONS

It will be useful to define three terms as they are used in this chapter.

Completed suicide means an act by which an individual has intentionally killed himself.

Attempted suicide refers to an act deliberately carried out by an individual against himself, by which he intends to endanger or end his life, or to give the appearance of such an intent, but which does not result in death. In many attempted suicides, the patient has conflicting feelings, simultaneously having a wish to live and a wish to die. In some instances, the death wish appears to be minimal, there being some other primary motivation, such as the manipulation of a spouse or the seeking of help. These have sometimes been referred to as suicidal gestures but are here included in the category of attempted suicide.

Potential suicide refers to the individual who, while not having made an attempt on his life, is thought to be in danger of doing so.

COMPLETED SUICIDES

In the United States, the rate of recorded suicides is about 11 per 100,000 persons per year.[3,11] An unknown number of suicides go unrecorded, death being wrongly attributed to other causes. Among completed suicides the ratio of men to women is between 2 to 1 and 4 to 1 throughout the industrialized world. In men, the suicide rate increases with age until the mid-80s and in women it peaks between ages 55 and 65. The suicide rate is substantially higher among single persons, particularly the widowed and divorced, than among the married. The rate is higher among whites than blacks and somewhat higher among Protestants than Jews and Catholics.

Most persons who have committed suicide have made previous attempts or have threatened to attempt suicide or both. Retrospective studies indicate that most completed suicides occur in people who have a psychiatric illness, depression being the most common diagnosis made in this group.[10] Persons afflicted with incurable or fatal physical illness account for a small fraction of completed suicides.

Of great significance is the fact that most persons who have died by suicide have a history of having consulted their physician within a year prior to death. Murphy found that of 32 persons who committed suicide

77

by overdose of medication, 29 (91 percent) had consulted one or more physicians within 6 months or less of their deaths.[8,9] Further, 16 of these patients (50 percent) had obtained lethal quantities of hypnotic medication in a single prescription and in most instances the prescription had been filled within 2 weeks of the suicide. In the same study it was found that of 28 persons who suicided by means other than overdose of medication, 20 (71 percent) had consulted their physician within 6 months of death. In both groups of suicides, the physician last seen was not a psychiatrist in 75 percent of the cases. In the same study it was noted that there was substantial evidence of depressive illness in three-quarters of the patients who had been seen by physicians but that the depressive illness was usually not diagnosed and therefore was rarely treated. The implications of these observations for suicide prevention are obvious. As Murphy points out, however, retrospective studies of completed suicides give no indication of the frequency with which physicians are successful in detection and management of suicidal risk.

THE POTENTIAL SUICIDAL RISK

Among both completed and attempted suicides, the most commonly made diagnosis is depression. Therefore, it is important to be alert to the presence of a depressive syndrome in any patient and, if found, to assess the suicidal risk and to institute treatment promptly. It is not uncommon for a depressed patient to focus primarily on physical symptoms and to "explain" his depressed mood as being secondary to them. In such cases, the diagnosis may be easily missed.

In the assessment of suicidal danger, it is useful to determine (1) the severity of depression, (2) the presence of hopelessness, (3) a prior history of suicide attempts, and (4) the presence of current suicidal thoughts and suicidal intentions.[2,7]

Severity of Depression   In the general adult population the occurrence of mild, transient periods of depressed mood is extremely high, perhaps universal. A depressive illness of significant severity exists if the mood disturbance has lasted for a month or longer and is accompanied by several or more of the following symptoms: insomnia; anorexia; weight loss (in absence of dieting or organic disease sufficient to account for loss of appetite and weight); fatigue; agitation; slowness of speech or activity; difficulty in concentrating; loss of interest; impotence; or feelings of guilt, inadequacy, unworthiness, or hopelessness and a wish to die.

In persons suffering from affective disorders, the lifetime risk of suicide has been estimated to be 15 percent.[4] Although there are numerous exceptions, there is some correlation between severity of depression and suicidal risk. Paradoxically, however, apparent symptomatic improvement in the course of the illness does not necessarily mean that the risk of suicide has decreased. Some patients may seem to have improved because they have secretly made a decision to commit suicide while others, who had been functionally incapacitated by severe depression, may become better able to carry out a suicide plan as their depression begins to lift.

Hopelessness   The patient who feels that his future is bleak, his problems insoluble, his illness incurable, that he is not worthy of relief, or worthy of any other good fortune represents a greater suicidal risk than does a person who, though depressed, has a hopeful outlook regarding his future. A hopeful, but nonetheless depressed, patient may make casual reference to future plans thus implying that he intends to be around.

Prior History of Suicide Attempts   A history of previous suicide attempts increases the probability of another attempt.

Verbalization of Suicidal Thoughts and Intent   A common error in dealing with a suspected suicidal patient is that of failing to ask him directly about his wishes and intentions regarding death and suicide. It is likely that all depressed patients, at one time or another, feel a wish to die and have thoughts of suicide. However, it is important directly to ask the patient if he has been preoccupied with death and suicidal thoughts and if he has, in the present or recently, actually intended to commit suicide. If he says he has so intended, the patient should also be asked to describe the method contemplated, whether he has procured the means to carry out the act, and other details.

The potentially suicidal patient may have an illness other than primary depression. In fact, any condition or situation that has resulted in a feeling of hopelessness may be associated with the danger of suicide. For example, persons confronted with public exposure of unethical behavior or evidence of incompetence, or individuals with progressive, incurable disease may choose death in preference to a future which they perceive as laden with unbearable misery. The schizophrenic patient may attempt suicide in a moment of despair or in response to an hallucinated command. The delirious patient, while not necessarily intending suicide, may seriously or fatally injure himself in a variety of ways, such as leaving the room via a window. The presence of alcoholism, especially if associated with depressive illness, increases the risk of suicide.

Management   The management of the suicidal patient consists of taking those steps necessary to protect him from self-destructive impulses and of treating the associated illness, usually depression, which is causing the patient to be suicidal. The practical importance of effective management of the suicidal patient is underscored by the fact that in most cases the patient remains actively intent upon suicide for only a limited period of time, eg, until there has been alleviation of the feeling of hopelessness. On the other hand, it may be impossible to prevent suicide by the person who keeps his despair and suicidal intent secret, or who persists in intention for suicide in spite of efforts to assist him with his emotional problems, or who suddenly acts on impulse.

If the physician has judged that there is grave and imminent risk of suicide (such as in the case of a depressed patient who feels hopeless or who is preoccupied with suicidal thoughts), he should discuss this openly with the patient and his next of kin. Psychiatric consultation should be obtained without delay. If psychiatric consultation is not immediately obtainable or if the circumstances otherwise warrant it, the physician may decide upon immediate hospitalization and institution of suicidal observation. The latter consists of the patient being constantly accompanied by a responsible person until the danger of suicide is considered to have abated. In addition, environmental opportunities for self-destruction are reduced to a minimum. This includes the provision of an unbreakable, locked window and the removal of objects, including medicine, with which the patient may harm himself. In severe depression requiring psychiatric hospitalization, electroconvulsive treatment may be indicated if the suicidal risk is judged to be especially grave or if the depression does not respond to chemotherapy and psychotherapy.

In many instances, the primary physician or the treating psychiatrist elects to treat the depressed person on an outpatient basis. This is done when the suicidal risk, though not entirely absent, is thought not to be overwhelming or imminent. Treatment with one of the tricyclic antidepressants in combination with supportive psychotherapy is usually indicated for depressive illness of moderate severity. In the outpatient management of depression it is wise to avoid the use of barbiturates or other potentially dangerous hypnotics and to manage the insomnia by administering most or all of the tricyclic antidepressants in the evening. If a hypnotic is necessary, flurazepam (Dalmane), or some other mild hypnotic which is relatively unlikely to be lethal if taken in overdose, may be used. It is of course unwise to attempt to bolster the mood of the depressed patient by cheerfully telling him that everything will be fine or by some other superficial "reassurance," for this is apt to create a feeling of not being understood and thus only add to the patient's despair. It is helpful, however, to let the patient know (1) that the physician realizes how real is the suffering of depression; (2) that often there are moments when any depressed patient doubts that he will ever feel well again; (3) that though the patient may have doubts about it, experience shows the chances for remission of the depression are very good; and (4) there is apt to be a "lag period" between initiating treatment and the beginning of substantial improvement.

THE SUICIDE ATTEMPT

In addition to the immediate medical or surgical management necessitated by the attempt itself, the physician must assess the seriousness of suicidal intent. To assist him in carrying out this assessment it is advisable, for both clinical and legal reasons, to obtain the assistance of a psychiatric consultant.

It would be impractical and probably unwise routinely to advise psychiatric hospitalization in every case of attempted suicide. The incidence of attempted suicide is conservatively estimated to be more than ten times that of completed suicide.[12] In contrast to the latter group, the rate of attempted suicide is higher among women than men and reaches its peak in the third decade of life. These statistical differences, coupled with the fact that most completed suicides have made previous attempts, suggest that the attempted suicide group is a heterogeneous one that partially contains those who will eventually compose the completed group, ie, as the attempted suicide group grows older it contributes substantially to those who complete suicide. It has been estimated that the risk of suicide in the attempted group is approximately 1 to 2 percent per year.

In assessing suicidal danger, the same principles apply which were discussed in the preceding section. In addition, it is helpful to take into account (1) the lethality of the attempt, (2) the circumstances surrounding the attempt, (3) precipitating factors, and (4) consequences.

Lethality of the Attempt   Lethality of the attempt refers to the danger to life posed by the act itself regardless of any mitigating circumstances. For example, the ingestion of a large number of barbiturate capsules and self-inflicted gunshot wounds to the head or chest are highly lethal acts, whereas an overdose of chlordiazepoxide and superficial lacerations are not. If the attempt is judged to be highly lethal, ie, if death probably would have ensued in the absence of timely intervention, it is best to presume that the suicidal intent was extremely serious and remains so in the immediate postattempt period. This is a practical policy even though it is recognized that an occasional patient may not be aware of the relative dangerousness of one type of attempt as opposed to another, eg, the lethality of barbiturate versus chlordiazepoxide overdosage. Obviously, the converse is not true. Low lethality does not necessarily point to low seriousness of intent.

Surrounding Circumstances   The following circumstances are positively correlated with seriousness of intent: (1) being alone at time of attempt; (2) actively taking precautions against being discovered; (3) the rescue of the patient could not reasonably have been foreseen by the patient; and (4) evidence of premeditation such as a suicide note, recent increase in life insurance, recently written will, or deliberate acquisition of material or equipment specifically needed for the attempt.

Precipitating Factors   The attempt may have arisen out of hopelessness and despair as part of a depressive illness or in association with some other illness or life situation. Not infrequently, however, the patient makes a suicide attempt, even a dangerous one, in order to bring about a change in his life situation. For example, the attempt may well be a "cry for help," an effort to arouse sympathetic concern by others or to change the direction in which an important relationship has been going. The attempt may be designed to punish someone, symbolically or actually, by evoking guilt. It may be an attempt to punish oneself.

It is, therefore, important to review with the patient what was going on in his life and in his mind at the time of the attempt. The patient should be asked if he had felt that the attempt would result in death. Had he thought that he might live, but that his life would be different? If so, how? Had he been angry and wanting to "get even" with someone? Had he felt guilty and that he deserved to be punished? Had he wanted to die?

Consequences   A key question is: does it appear that the suicide attempt will be followed by significant changes in the patient or in his circumstances? If the physician has been able to gauge the patient's original purposes, feelings, and expectations prior to the attempt, he may be able to ascertain the psychologic and interpersonal results of the attempt. For example, if one infers that the patient had sought to be less isolated, to be more accepted by family, to get help for his problems or his depression, does the attempt promise to succeed in his substantially achieving these goals? Does the patient seem unsurprised, perhaps even glad, that he is still alive? Does he seem to feel less guilty than before the attempt? Did the suicide attempt achieve nothing as far as the patient is concerned? Does he now feel even less adequate and more isolated than before? Did he "wake up" to find a sullen, resentful spouse and an emergency room staff too harried with "real" emergencies to be very concerned with him?

All of the above categories of factors have to be weighed in forming a decision as to the seriousness of intent and the continuing danger of suicide.

Management   It is prudent to obtain psychiatric consultation and to institute suicidal precautions until psychiatric evaluation indicates that this is no longer necessary. The essential principles of management are the same as those discussed in the preceding section. It is often and properly decided that the patient who has made a suicide attempt does not require psychiatric hospitalization. In that event, it is mandatory to recommend outpatient psychiatric observation and treatment. Unfortunately, a substantial percentage of suicide attempters for whom psychiatric treatment has been arranged fail to keep their appointments or drop out of treatment prematurely. This fact underscores the importance of thoroughly discussing the need for treatment with the patient and with important members of his family.

ACUTE BEHAVIORAL DISTURBANCES

Often, the patient who engages in aggressive, inappropriate, bizarre, or otherwise disturbing behavior does not seek medical attention on his own initiative because he is either unaware of the pathology of his behavior or is unconcerned about it, or both. Therefore, he frequently comes to medical attention at the behest of a concerned member of the family or a friend. Because of the patient's own lack of insight into his condition, the concerned relative may be perplexed as to "how to get him to the doctor" and may decide upon some sort of deceptive ruse such as telling the patient that he himself needs to see the physician and wishes to have the patient accompany him. It is unwise for the physician to go along with any subterfuge designed to trick the patient into seeing the doctor, for the loss of trust resulting from such a deception will often make further work with the patient impossible. The family should be advised to discuss the patient's condition directly, but gently, with him and firmly to insist upon the necessity of medical examination.

Acute behavioral disturbances may be characterized by one or more of the following: (1) recent development of behavior that is "out of character" for the patient such as acting impulsively, showing poor judgment, or seeming to be unresponsive, distant, uncaring; (2) aggressive or violent behavior; (3) excessive activity, verbal or nonverbal; (4) inactivity, withdrawal; (5) bizarre, silly, or "crazy" behavior; and (6) behavior characterized by evidence of confusion or amnesia.

It is essential to have the best informed and most responsible members of the family accompany the patient to the place of examination. If the preexamination contact with the family indicates that there may be a problem in controlling the patient's behavior, it is wise to arrange for the examination to be in the hospital emergency room or other suitable location rather than in one's private office. The examination of the patient should include a mental status examination and a careful physical and neurologic examination as soon as the patient's behavior permits.

THE VIOLENT PATIENT

Although the diagnostic considerations that arise in the evaluation of violent behavior do not essentially differ from those of other kinds of disturbing behavior, the violent patient does require that certain immediate steps be taken. As with acute anxiety or panic, diagnosis and therapeutic management go hand-in-hand.

The excited, threatening, or combative patient instills fear in everyone in contact with him, including the physician. As Lion points out, it is useful to assume that the violent patient is afraid of losing control of his own aggressive impulses.[5,6] Thus, the physician has two immediate objectives. First, he should establish verbal contact with the patient and reassure him that he will be effectively helped to control his aggression, that he will not be allowed to translate his feelings into destructive behavior. Second, he should encourage the patient to talk freely about his current feelings including his fears and anger. This is done not with the objective of getting the patient to reveal what precipitated his disturbance but simply to help him substitute verbalization of feelings for action.

An excited, belligerent patient will often begin to grow calmer as the physician quietly explains that he wishes to help the patient, that he would like to talk with him about his feelings and problems, and offers the patient an opportunity to be interviewed alone. However, if the physician is fearful for his own safety, he should not make such an offer but instead talk with the patient in the presence of two or three attendants or in a room with the door open and with assistants standing nearby. The presence of several assistants may in itself help to calm the patient who fears loss of control.

The focus of the interview should be primarily upon the patient's current feelings and thoughts. It is important to avoid promising the patient not to hospitalize him. The physician should simply indicate that the objective is to try to understand the patient's feelings and that the interviewer and his staff will help him to avoid loss of control of his impulses or angry feelings. In the initial stages of the evaluation, it is wise not to probe into the circumstances or issues which may have precipitated the rage, since this may provoke exacerbation. Such exploration, while important, can be done later. For example, if one suspects that the rage is covering homosexual panic, it would be unwise to "fish" for material to support that hypothesis.

Occasionally the excited, violent patient will not respond to the approach described above or will be too disturbed to allow the physician to attempt such an approach. In this event, physical constraints are necessary. The application of them, such as devices to immobilize the patient's arms and legs, should be done by several attendants under the supervision of the physician. Once the patient is restrained on a stretcher or bed, the administration of a suitable drug is often indicated. Chlorpromazine, 50 to 100 mg intramuscularly, may be given and repeated hourly until control is obtained. In an elderly patient, or a patient in whom there is special need to reduce possible hypotensive side effects, a benzodiazepine may be preferred: 50 to 100 mg of chlordiazepoxide intramuscularly or 10 to 20 mg of diazepam intramuscularly may be given and repeated hourly as necessary. Vital signs, including blood pressure, should be frequently monitored. Haloperidol, which is somewhat less sedating and has less hypotensive effect than chlorpromazine, may be administered in doses of 4 to 6 mg intramuscularly and may be repeated once or twice at hourly intervals if necessary.

DIAGNOSTIC EVALUATION OF ACUTE BEHAVIORAL DISTURBANCES

As enumerated above, from a descriptive viewpoint, a variety of behavior patterns may alarm the patient and family and prompt them to seek immediate medical attention. A useful diagnostic approach is to determine if the acute behavioral disturbance is (1) organic or (2) functional, and then to proceed toward a more specific diagnostic entity.

(1) In general, acute disturbances of behavior in which organic factors play a major etiologic role are associated with evidence of impaired intellectual functions such as one or more of the following: disorientation, memory impairment, difficulty in comprehension and abstract thinking, rambling and incoherent speech, and drowsiness. In the hallucinating patient, a predominance of visual hallucinations favors an organic basis although it may be a feature of early, acutely developing schizophrenic decompensation.

Careful review of the alcohol and drug history is extremely important because of the frequency of intoxication and withdrawal syndromes. The type of drug or drugs, dosage, frequency of usage, and length of time since last dose are essential data for diagnosis and management. History of abusing one drug should arouse suspicion that other drugs also have been taken, knowingly or unknowingly. There may be associated physical signs such as pinpoint pupils, slow respiration, venous thrombosis and scarring in opioid intoxication; dilated pupils, flushed and dry skin, urinary retention in intoxication with atropinelike drugs; tremulousness, sweating, restlessness, and seizures in withdrawal from barbiturates or other CNS depressants; goose flesh, yawning, rhinorrhea, abdominal cramps in opioid withdrawal; drowsiness, slurred speech, and ataxia in intoxication with alcohol and other CNS depressant drugs.

Other aspects of the medical history also must be carefully reviewed. In addition to drug intoxication and withdrawal, organic brain syndromes may be associated with head trauma, metabolic disorders, febrile condi tions, and any intracranial or systemic disease that alters cerebral structure and/or function. A history of "spells" or repeated, discrete episodes of behavioral disturbance, with or without amnesia, especially if associated with automatic or stereotyped behavior, olfactory hallucinations, micropsia, or macropsia, should arouse suspicion of seizure disorder.

Evidence in favor of an organic condition may indicate a variety of diagnostic procedures such as prompt chemical determinations of blood and urine, skull x-ray, EEG, and repeated neurologic examinations.

(2) Functional disturbances are usually not associated with the type of intellectual impairment that produces defective recent memory and disorientation. Careful examination and judgment, however, may be required in order to determine that the patient has a clear sensorium. For example, the schizophrenic patient may give a bizarre response when asked to state where he is though later indicating, in response to a more oblique inquiry, that he is clearly aware of his location. The severely depressed patient, or any patient who is self-absorbed and preoccupied, may appear to have a poor memory for recent events. For example, he may not recall what he had for breakfast because he was too preoccupied for it to have registered.

Most functional behavioral emergencies are associated with schizophrenic, manic, hysteric, or situational disturbances. The diagnostic characteristics of these conditions will be described in later chapters.

The importance of careful examination in making a psychiatric diagnosis is illustrated by the following case.

A young adult woman was rushed by ambulance to the hospital in the company of her acutely worried husband. Two hours before her arrival, she experienced the rapid onset of paralysis of the legs. Hurried examination in the emergency room revealed complete paralysis of both legs, marked weakness of the arms, and total anesthesia from the level of the umbilicus to the toes. Within an hour, the upper level of anesthesia had moved upward to the level of the thyroid cartilage. Her respirations were rapid but shallow. In anticipation of respiratory embarrassment, an emergency tracheotomy was done; this procedure was accomplished without administration of a local anesthetic since the incision was made below the upper level of anesthesia produced by the patient's illness. Following tracheotomy, the patient was transported by stretcher to the floor where she was to receive respiratory assistance as needed. On her way to the floor, the patient regained use of her extremities and the anesthesia markedly receded. The original examining physician subsequently recalled that during the paralysis and anesthesia, all tendon reflexes were present and plantar responses flexor. The diagnosis was conversion hysteria.

Although this case is unusually dramatic it is not uncommon for hysterical patients to have surgical procedures done to themselves.

It is wise to obtain prompt psychiatric consultation in all cases of acute behavioral disturbance, including those in which an organic component is strongly suspected.

If the acute behavioral disturbance is based upon an organic condition, hospitalization is mandatory in order to safely manage the patient while the specific nature of the organic or toxic factors is being determined. The patient's behavior may necessitate the temporary use of chemotherapeutic agents in order to allow further examination to proceed. Delirious patients must be carefully observed. Confusion and the likelihood of panic can be reduced, especially at night, by keeping the room well lighted when the patient is awake, having a trained person in constant attendance, addressing the patient in clear, simple terms, and otherwise avoiding ambiguous environmental cues.

Usually it is also wise to hospitalize the patient with acute functional psychosis. However, if such a patient is not suicidal or homocidal, responds well to the intramuscular administration of antipsychotic agents while under observation for a period of several hours, and has one or more responsible relatives to care for him, it may be feasible to offer psychiatric treatment in an outpatient setting in which he is seen initially on a daily basis.

Special Cases   We have discussed emergency situations arising from acute behavioral disturbances. Occasionally, however, a chronically ill patient may present a type of emergency because of the particular life circumstances in which his illness developed. For example, the patient with an organic brain syndrome, even in the absence of an acute disturbance of behavior, requires immediate, active management if he is a practicing physician or is in any other position in which the welfare of others is gravely jeopardized by the effects of his illness.

PANIC

Regardless of their cause, all states of acute, severe anxiety or panic are characterized by intense fear, restlessness, and various other symptoms and signs such as palpitations, a feeling of suffocating, blurring of vision, tachycardia, pallor, and sweating. Commonly, the patient's fear becomes localized or specific such as fear of death through suffocation or cardiac arrest, or of going crazy. Sometimes the source of danger is projected onto the external world.

The most common conditions associated with panic are (1) anxiety neurosis, (2) a "bad trip" with an hallucinogenic agent, (3) the acute phase of a schizophrenic illness (including homosexual panic), (4) amphetamine or cocaine intoxication, and (5) delirium.

Diagnostic and therapeutic management of the acute attack must be done in parallel. Having established the presence of acute anxiety, the physician should matter-of-factly discuss that fact with the patient. While acknowledging the patient's extreme discomfort, he should reassure him about specific fears, eg, that his condition will not cause his heart to stop and that his fearfulness itself has momentarily affected his judgment. Usually, a neurotic patient will respond to sympathetic attention, reassurance, and an opportunity to discuss his feelings with the physician; in the process of symptomatic abatement, it becomes evident that he manifests no evidence of psychosis. In anxiety neurosis, the patient may have a history of previous attacks.

If the panic state is part of a psychotic condition, the patient does not usually respond to psychologic support as readily as does the neurotic patient. As a general rule, acute schizophrenic illness and amphetamine intoxication are associated with a clear sensorium. The latter closely simulates paranoid schizophrenia and can only be diagnosed with confidence by obtaining a history of excessive amphetamine ingestion. The "bad trip" resulting from ingestion of an hallucinogen may be associated with extreme anxiety. The patient will often reveal his drug history, particularly if the importance of doing so is explained to him. He may or may not be disoriented. Delirium may be associated with extreme fear.

MANAGEMENT

Psychiatric consultation should be obtained. Chemotherapeutic intervention is often necessary in panic associated with psychosis, whether functional or toxic. The choice of drug is based upon considerations similar to those mentioned in management of the violent patient and will be discussed further in Chapters 10, 12, 15, and 18. Phenothiazines are usually not employed in treating intoxication with hallucinogenic substances. If the anxiety state is associated with an organic or toxic psychosis, hospitalization is indicated. In the event of functional psychosis, the decision to hospitalize is based upon the same factors discussed in the management of acute behavioral disturbances.

REFERENCES

1. Anderson WH, Kuehnle JC: Strategies for the treatment of acute psychosis. JAMA 229:1884, 1974

2. Beck AT, Resnik HLP, Jettieri DH: The Prediction of Suicide. Bowie, Md, Charles Press, 1974
3. Dublin L: Suicide: A Sociological and Statistical Study. New York, Ronald Press, 1963
4. Guze SB, Robins R: Suicide and primary affective disorders. Br J Psychiat 117:437, 1970
5. Lion JR: Evaluation and Management of the Violent Patient. Springfield, Ill, Thomas, 1972
6. Lion JR, Azcarate C, Christopher R, Arana JD: A violence clinic. Md State Med J 23:45, 1974
7. Minkoff M, Bergman E, Beck AT, Beck R: Hopelessness, depression, and attempted suicide. Am J Psychiat 130:455, 1973
8. Murphy GE: The physician's responsibility for suicide. I. an error of commission. Ann Intern Med 82:301, 1975
9. Murphy GE: The physician's responsibility of suicide. II. errors of omission. Ann Intern Med 82:301, 1975
10. Robins E, Gassner S, Kayes J, et al: The communication of suicidal intent. A study of 134 consecutive cases of successful (completed) suicide. Am J Psychiat 115:724, 1959
11. Schneidman ES: Suicide. In Freedman AM, Kaplan HJ, Sadock BJ (eds): Comprehensive Textbook of Psychiatry, 2nd ed. Baltimore, Williams and Wilkins, 1975, pp 1774-85
12. Weissman MM: The epidemology of suicide attempts, 1960-1971. Arch Gen Psychiat 30:737, 1974

Chapter

8

Sexual Dysfunction

In recent years, sexual behavior has received a great deal of attention in both professional and lay circles. Indeed it has been said that a "revolution" has occurred in the Western world, particularly in the United States, in attitudes toward and mores concerning sexual behavior. People have become "liberated" in the sense that they are freer to talk and write about sex and perhaps to engage in sexual behavior, in or out of marriage, than was the case in their parents' and grandparents' times. This liberation doubtlessly stems from several factors, among them the widespread availability of "the pill" and the Zeitgeist of the mid-20th century with its almost obsessional emphasis on freedom of expression, sexual and otherwise.

This new-found sexual freedom has not, of course, eradicated disorders of sexual function, but it does seem to have contributed to a greater readiness on the part of individuals and couples to recognize sexual problems and to seek help for them. The pioneering and widely publicized work of Masters and Johnson has significantly contributed to our understanding of normal sexual functioning and to the understanding and management of sexual disorders.[4,5] In view of these changes in society's attitude toward sex and the widely recognized effectiveness of "sex therapy," it is to be expected that patients will frequently consult their family physician about sexual problems believing that he will be able to help them or refer them to specialists in this field.

SOME BASIC FEATURES OF HUMAN SEXUALITY

Like other aspects of human behavior, sexual functioning is determined by a combination of hereditary or constitutional factors on the one hand and environmental or experiential ones on the other.

SEXUAL IDENTITY AND GENDER ROLE

Anatomic or biologic sexual identity as male or female is determined by the individual's chromosomal complement, XX for the female and XY for the male, with corresponding male and female genital and gonadal development. A rare but important exception is seen in the testicular feminization or androgen insensitivity syndrome characterized by XY chromosomes, undescended testicles, female external genitalia, female secondary sexual characteristics, and female gender role. Persons with this syndrome are women in terms of psychologic identification and social role.

As a rule, gender role matches anatomic sex. This is to be expected since the rearing persons take their cue from the anatomic sex of the infant in assigning the role of male or female to him or her. However, for reasons that are not entirely clear, there may on rare occasions be a disparity between anatomic sex and gender role development resulting in transsexualism or gender role dysphoria; this is often a painfully conflictful state which leads the individual to seek treatment in the form of psychotherapy and sometimes, if psychiatric treatment has failed, sex reassignment surgery. Gender role problems may also arise when congenital abnormalties of the external genitalia result in anatomic ambiguity and hence in gender assignment in infancy that proves to be inappropriate as the individual matures.

Psychosexual development cannot be divorced from the overall psychologic or emotional development of the individual. For example, a satisfying, fulfilled sexual life depends in part upon successful resolution of the oedipal stage of development with consequent freedom to relate to and love another individual as a truly separate person and not as a symbolic representation (substitute) of an infantile object choice. Neurotic conflicts regarding object choice, sexual fantasies, or one's own adequacy can seriously interfere with the development of intimate relationships and can lead to avoidance of sexual activity or to a reduction of sex to its purely physical components.

THE SEXUAL RESPONSE CYCLE

The sexual response cycle refers to the various stages of sexual response that occur in males and females in which orgasm is achieved. This was elucidated by Masters and Johnson.[5]

The first phase is that of excitement characterized by erection in the male and vaginal lubrication in the female. This is followed by the plateau phase characterized in the male by increased penile tumescence, contraction of the cremasteric muscles with consequent positioning of the testes close to the perineum, and in the female by further vascular engorgement and reddening of the labia minora. Orgasm is the third phase and in both sexes consists of a highly pleasurable, rapid release from the preceding sexual tension. In the male, the first stage of orgasm consists of an awareness of ejaculatory inevitability followed by urethral contraction and a sensation of semen moving through the urethra. In the female, orgasm begins with a momentary suspension of arousal followed by sensual radiations from the clitoris into the pelvis and a sensation of warmth spreading from the pelvic region to the rest of the body. Resolution or relaxation follows. In the male there occurs a refractory period in which further arousal and erection do not occur. Women do not have this refractory period and thus are capable of having several orgasms in succession.

This is a general outline of the sexual response cycle; there is much variation from one individual to another and within a given individual at various times. The rate of arousal and rate of passage from one phase to another can vary. In addition, not everyone has an orgasm each time. Knowing about these variations can help allay a patient's apprehensions about being abnormal. The mutual sharing of pleasuring and the intimate communication of sexual interest are more important than achieving some stereotypical norm of performance.

ASSESSMENT OF SEXUAL FUNCTIONING

The physician may discover the existence of sexual problems in several ways.[2,6] The patient may directly present with an overt complaint of sexual dysfunction, he may indirectly do so by presenting with symptomatic complaints that suggest the presence of sexual problems, and, finally, the physician may learn of the sexual problems in the course of routinely obtaining the sexual history.

Here it may be said that including an inquiry into the patient's sexual experiences as part of the initial, routine medical history is a way of letting the patient know that the physician is interested in and willing to help with sexual problems. This in itself may help the patient feel freer to bring up questions or concerns about his or his partner's sexual functioning.

In eliciting the sexual history (whether this is initiated by the physician or the patient) the physician uses a nonjudgmental, matter-of-fact approach. He does not shy away from asking relevant questions but does so in a respectful and tactful manner, one which takes the patient's sensitivity into account and which helps to allay tension or embarrassment. The physician must take care to use terms the patient understands, which sometimes is best done by using terms which the patient himself has introduced as long as their meaning is clear to both parties. In history taking it is always important to allow enough time so that one can unhurriedly listen to the patient's detailed description of his experiences and ask appropriate questions; this is particularly the case when sexual problems are being reviewed. Generally it is helpful initially to direct one's questions toward those areas which are least personal or least apt to arouse anxiety. When the physician suspects that the patient is troubled with feelings of embarrassment or inadequacy, he may make a casual comment which lets the patient know that many people have had the sort of experience or feeling or problem that he has.

When a sexual dysfunction problem has been presented or elicited, the physician proceeds to obtain a detailed history of its development. This should include the life situation concurrent with the onset, remissions, and exacerbations of the complaint. Particular attention should be paid to the quality of the emotional relationship between the patient and his or her sexual partner and to possible correlations between changes in that relationship and sexual functioning of both partners. Of considerable diagnostic importance is a history of situational variance in sexual functioning such as the presence of impotence or anorgasmia with one partner but not another or during attempted intercourse as compared with masturbation.

It was mentioned earlier that the patient may not complain openly of a sexual difficulty but may instead present with symptoms which are the byproduct of sexual dysfunction or which serve as a means of seeking help. Examples of such complaints include headaches, backaches, or some other discomfort which tend to occur in the evenings or on weekends when the spouse is at home, or which tend to remit when the spouse is away on a trip. Such indirect presentation may or may not pose considerable difficulties to the interviewer depending in part upon the degree to which the patient is consciously aware of the associated interpersonal and sexual problems. In the presence of considerable anxiety and defensiveness the physician approaches the issue at the level presented by the patient, eg, at first dealing with the physical symptoms, later broaching the interpersonal situations connected with the symptoms, and eventually the sexual aspects of the patient's problems. This approach often requires a number of interviews and the physician must be prepared to allow the patient to "retreat" to a nonanxiety topic, such as a physical complaint, when the patient's discomfort leads him or her to this type of defensive operation. This interviewing technique is also discussed in Chapter 16.

During the assessment process it is often extremely valuable to interview the patient's sexual partner separately or conjointly with the patient. This step of course can only be taken after it has been discussed with the patient and then only with the patient's consent and cooperation. When a couple is experiencing sexual difficulty, it is not uncommon for the individual whose sexual function is the least impaired to be the one who seeks help, since his or her self-esteem is less threatened than that of the more dysfunctional partner.[6]

It is of considerable importance in the planning of management to assess etiologic factors as far as is feasible to do so. Some sexual dysfunction problems appear to stem from lack of information or actual misinformation about sexual anatomy and physiology. In other instances, a current interpersonal problem or emotional difficulty such as depression may seem to be the primary issue of which the sexual dysfunction is but one manifestation. It is always important to make careful inquiry into alcohol and drug usage and to be alert to a history of physical illnesses such as diabetes which may interfere with sexual function. Sometimes a single instance of performance failure in males will give rise to fear of another failure sufficiently intense that performance is in fact blocked, a very unpleasant sort of self-fulfilling prophecy. Occasionally, sexual dysfunction arises from unconscious and deeply rooted psychologic conflict which is only approachable therapeutically by intensive psychotherapy.

The assessment of sexual dysfunction always includes a general medical evaluation to rule out organic processes which may interfere with sexual function.

COMMON SEXUAL PROBLEMS

The most common sexual problems which the primary physician is apt to see are those experienced by married couples.[3,4] It is difficult to define precisely what is good or adequate sexual function because what constitutes a satisfactory situation for one couple may be quite unsatisfactory for another. For most practical purposes sexual dysfunction refers to sexual functioning that is less than satisfactory for one or both members of the couple. It should be pointed out that even when the sexual dysfunction problem is clearly assigned to only one member of the couple, both members of the marital couple are involved, ie, both are affected by the disability, both will be affected by therapeutic outcome, in some instances both have contributed to etiology, and not uncommonly both may need to participate in the treatment process.

SEXUAL DYSFUNCTION IN MEN

The commonest sexual disorders in men are impotence, premature ejaculation, and retarded ejaculation.

Impotence   This refers to the inability to achieve an erection sufficient for penetration or to maintain an erection until intercourse is completed. (Completion of intercourse usually refers to ejaculation. However, older males not infrequently discontinue intercourse without having achieved ejaculation. The patient with retarded ejaculation may "give up" and discontinue intercourse because of discouragement or fatigue even though continuing to maintain penile erection.)

Most cases of impotence, at least in young and middle-aged males, are psychologically caused ("functional"), but organic causes must be ruled out. Impotence secondary to organic disease is usually characterized by complete impotence or progressively worsening impotence and the disability is relatively unaffected by situational factors. On the other hand, a history of being able to achieve an erection with one sexual partner but not another or during masturbation but not intercourse favors the diagnosis of functional disorder. Similarly, the occurrence of full and firm, nocturnal, full-bladder erections in an impotent male favors the functional diagnosis.

Ejaculatory Disorders   Premature ejaculation refers to the repeated experience in which ejaculation occurs during foreplay, at the time of penetration, or after only a few thrusts following intromission. This condition is almost always on a psychogenic basis although inflammatory, irritating conditions affecting the glands, prepuce, urethra, or prostate have been cited as possible contributing factors.

In retarded ejaculation the male finds it very difficult to achieve ejaculation or does not ejaculate at all during intercourse while usually being able to ejaculate by masturbation. This condition too is usually psychogenic but can be mimicked by retrograde ejaculation which may be associated with urologic procedures. Thioridazine administration may produce ejaculatory inhibition as may intoxication with CNS depressants such as alcohol.

SEXUAL DYSFUNCTION IN WOMEN

The most common types of sexual dysfunction in women are anorgasmia, dyspareunia, and vaginismus.

Anorgasmia   This condition is characterized by inability to experience orgasm despite apparently adequate stimulation. Some patients with this condition are unable to have orgasm during either coitus or masturbation. Others are able to achieve orgasm during masturbation only. This condition is seldom primarily caused by organic factors although physical illness, including gynecologic disorders, may provide a basis for anxious concern which interferes with the individual's freedom to function sexually.

Dyspareunia   Painful sensations which prevent coitus or make enjoyment of it impossible are commonly secondary to local pathology such as inflammatory conditions involving the vulva or vagina, torn uterine ligament, pelvic inflammatory disease, and endometriosis. These and other organic factors must be carefully excluded. A history of dyspareunia which is markedly affected by situational factors such as being present with one partner but not another supports the diagnosis of a psychogenic disorder.

Vaginismus   In this condition there is contraction of the pelvic musculature which renders penetration of the vagina difficult or impossible. Here too it is important that local physical disorders be excluded. Ability to function better under some circumstances as compared with others supports a functional diagnosis.

In addition to the above specific dysfunctions, one or both members of the marital couple may complain of a general decline in sexual interest, activity, and degree of satisfaction derived from their sexual relationship.

The source of the difficulty may be related to deficient sexual techniques but more often than not the problem arises from disturbance and conflict in the relationship between the two persons. Occasionally, of course, the loss of interest by one partner may be accompanied by an extramarital affair with all of the complications which may be associated with that situation.

MANAGEMENT [3,4,6]

The management of sexual dysfunction is determined by careful assessment of those factors which have contributed to etiology. As a general rule it is necessary to involve both members of the couple in the therapy.

If during a thorough review of the couple's sexual history, the physician has concluded that one or both of them lack basic information about sexual functioning, and that this lack has contributed to faulty techniques and/or inappropriate expectations, the physician may adopt what is basically an educational or information-giving approach. This approach of course must be carried out in a respectful, unhurried fashion, usually over a period of several office visits, and with due attention to the possibility that problems other than lack of information may be contributing to the couple's difficulty. A decade ago there was a commonly held myth (perhaps disseminated by alleged experts on sex) that the truly well-adjusted couple regularly experienced simultaneous orgasms. One of the present authors heard a well-known therapist confidently assert to a mixed audience that there is no such thing as a frigid woman, only inadequate men! However, most persons who are uninformed or misinformed about sexual matters may be so because they have been somehow personally inhibited from learning about this aspect of life, perhaps because of early environmental influences. It is not unusual for the man to be more or less unaware of the importance of foreplay because he is apt to reach the stage of arousal far more quickly than does his partner. Neither party may have thought it of much importance to learn what is particularly pleasurable to his or her partner. Through engaging the couple in discussions of their sexual experiences the physician has an opportunity not only to supply information and correct distortions but also to convey to the couple that sexual function is a legitimate topic in which to be interested, and that they can learn from each other if they are willing to communicate.

A common experience of men who are impotent is that fear of failure actively interferes with performance. With anorgasmic women there is often an inhibition of enjoyment of physical, sensuous stimuli and a self-defeating overemphasis on the goal of achieving orgasm to the exclusion of simply enjoying the sexual experience. In the Masters–Johnson approach, or one of its modifications, the couple is instructed to engage in activities in which they give each other pleasure through kissing, petting, and caressing, but to avoid genital contact. The latter prohibition removes the fear of failure and counteracts excessive emphasis upon the goal of orgasm. The vicious circle of failure and tension is thus broken. After a period of mutual pleasuring, the couple is instructed to include genital touching and caressing and eventually are led by graded exercises to sexual intercourse. In the case of premature ejaculation a special technique, the "squeeze" technique, can be used. This allows the man to have relatively prolonged experiences with sexual play and eventually coitus before he ejaculates.

In those instances in which it is judged that a simple educational approach is not sufficient and that a Masters–Johnson type of treatment approach is indicated, the physician should refer the patient to a psychiatrist or some other specialist who has had experiences in treating sexual disorders.

Not uncommonly, sexually dysfunctional couples have difficulties in their relationship with each other, of which the sexual dysfunction is one manifestation. For this reason, it is the usual practice for the therapist(s) to engage the couple in exploration of their feelings, attitudes, and behavior toward each other, and to supplement the more mechanical aspects of sexual therapy with counseling for interpersonal difficulties. It is not rare for sexual dysfunction in one or both members of the couple to be based on deeply rooted, unconscious conflict. When this is the case more intensive psychoanalytically oriented psychotherapy or psychoanalysis is indicated.

THE PARAPHILIAS

The paraphilias include a variety of sexual behaviors which may or may not be looked upon as abnormal or as constituting a problem by the individual who engages in the behavior. Included in the paraphilias are the following.

SEXUAL ORIENTATION DISTURBANCE

This refers to homosexuality about which the individual is anxious or in conflict. Not infrequently the practicing homosexual is content with his or her sexual orientation. Sometimes, however, the overtly homosexual person is seriously troubled because he or she wishes to be married some day and have a family or, in the event that the person is already married, has encountered serious difficulty in the sexual relationship with the spouse. Strong homosexual inclinations which are unconscious constitute latent homosexuality and may set the stage for homosexual panic if strong homosexual feelings erupt into consciousness. Mild or fleeting feelings of attraction to persons of the same sex are not uncommon among psychologically healthy adults.

SEXUAL DEVIATIONS

Sexual deviation refers to a group of sexual behaviors which includes sadomasochism, pedophilia, fetishism, voyeurism, exhibitionism, and transvestism. Incest is also included in this category. These behavior problems are symptoms of serious emotional disturbance. In some instances, the sexual behavior poses a threat to others and may require legal as well as therapeutic intervention.

GENDER DYSPHORIA SYNDROME

In this syndrome the individual, male or female, is markedly discontented with the gender role corresponding to his or her anatomic sex. The patient may dress in clothes belonging to the opposite sex not for sexual excitement or pleasure as with the transvestite but because of a desire to live as a member of the opposite sex.

Management of the patient with one of the paraphilias requires referral to a psychiatrist or a sexual therapy clinic specializing in the evaluation and treatment of these and other sexual disorders.

SEXUAL PROBLEMS ASSOCIATED WITH PHYSICAL ILLNESS

Patients with chronic illnesses and those recovering from acute illnesses such as myocardial infarction usually want to continue or resume sexual activity. In most instances they can and should do so. In all patients it is obviously desirable that resumption of sexual activity be a planned part of medical management so that anxiety related to performance capability or to the physical effect of sexual activity can be minimized.

After recovery from a myocardial infarction, men can usually resume sexual activity commensurate with their tolerance of other physical exercise. Though there is a myth that postcoronary men have a high risk of dying during intercourse, this is actually a rare occurrence. There does seem to be some risk associated with who the man's sexual partner is rather than the fact of having intercourse. The stress of coitus with a new partner, as in an extramarital affair, is evidently more risky than intercourse with the marital partner.[7]

In discussing sexual activity with a man recovering from a coronary, his recent and present level of activity should be ascertained. Graded exercises under the supervision of a physiotherapist is often useful in rehabilitation of the patient. When the patient is able to tolerate such exercise as climbing two flights of stairs, he can begin to use this exercise capacity for sexual activity. It may be advisable for the patient to resume sexual activity gradually rather than all at once, eg, petting, perhaps masturbation, then intercourse. In intercourse he might use a position other than male superior, since the isometric contraction of arm and shoulder muscles in this position is strenuous.[7]

Diabetes can be a cause of impotence due to autonomic nervous system degeneration; this is generally irreversible. Occasionally the impotence improves with better control of the diabetes. More commonly, though, the man so afflicted will have to replace intercourse with other sexual activities. If the couple are still interested in having a sex life, they may try oral and manual techniques; although the man cannot have a full erection he may still be able to have orgasm.

Paraplegia and arthritis cause reduction of motility. In addition, the paraplegic has little or no sensory input that he is aware of from the genital area. Nonetheless, reflex activity at the spinal cord level can lead to a firm erection, and paraplegics can derive pleasure from sexual activity. Helping the patient to be aware of this potential should be part of his rehabilitation program. The general approach to helping paraplegics and other patients with neuromuscular or musculoskeletal disabilities includes good communication between sexual partners, and experimentation and innovation with feasible positions and techniques.[2]

Hysterectomy can be followed by sexual difficulties for a couple.[8] The woman may become depressed after this surgery, and either she or her spouse may believe that hysterectomy signifies loss of sexuality or femininity. Counseling before and after surgery is wise; it may prevent some problems entirely and can greatly limit the severity of others.

ALTERED SEXUAL FUNCTIONING ASSOCIATED WITH MEDICATIONS

The historic quest for true aphrodisiacs is an ancient one indeed and it would appear that in every age there have been false claims and rumors of agents that enhance libido and ability to perform. Our age is no exception. In general, the efficacy of drugs in enhancing sexual interest and activity is not very impressive.[1]

Some agents such as alcohol, amphetamines, hallucinogens, and cannabis in low to moderate amounts may transiently produce an apparent increase in sexual interest and activity by decreasing inhibitions. Cannabis, amphetamines, hallucinogens, and cocaine may also be associated

100

with a heightened awareness of sensual experiences. However, these effects are difficult to measure, many reports of drug effects are anecdotal, and it is difficult to rule out placebo effect in many instances. The administration of L-dopa to patients with parkinsonism is sometimes associated with increased sexual activity; this may be due in part to overall improvement in the patient's condition.

In contrast with the relative ineffectiveness of drugs in improving sexual function, a number of agents can clearly have an adverse effect on sexual desire, potency, and ejaculation. Long-term addiction to heroin, morphine, and the barbiturates frequently produces a marked decline in sexual interest. Some decrease in libido may also be observed with the use of antipsychotic drugs, especially when employed in high doses.

Impotence can occur with the use of alcohol in large amounts, the phenothiazines, and sometimes with anticholinergic agents.

A small percentage of patients receiving thioridazine (Mellaril) report absence of ejaculate which is probably due to retrograde ejaculation. Premature ejaculation is commonly present following withdrawal from opiates in persons addicted to them.

REFERENCES

1. Carter CS, Davis JM: Effects of drugs on sexual arousal and performance. In Meyer JK (ed): Clinical Management of Sexual Disorders. Baltimore, Williams and Wilkins, 1976
2. Green R (ed): Human Sexuality, A Health Practitioner's Text. Baltimore, Williams and Wilkins, 1975
3. Levine SB: Marital sexual dysfunction. Introductory concepts. Ann Intern Med 84:448, 1976
4. Masters WH, Johnson VE: Human Sexual Inadequacy. Boston, Little, Brown, 1970
5. Masters WH, Johnson VE: Human Sexual Response. Boston, Little, Brown, 1966
6. Meyer JK (ed): Clinical Management of Sexual Disorders. Baltimore, Williams and Wilkins, 1976
7. Wagner NN: Sexual activity and the cardiac patient. In Green R (ed): Human Sexuality, A Health Practitioner's Text. Baltimore, Williams and Wilkins, 1975
8. Wolf S: Emotional reactions to hysterectomy. Postgrad Med 47:165, 1970

Chapter

9

Alcoholism

Pontine Myelinolysis
Diagnosis and Management
Alcoholism
    DIAGNOSIS
    MANAGEMENT
Alcohol Intoxication
Pathologic Intoxication
Withdrawal Syndromes
    DELIRIUM TREMENS

Alcoholism is a chronic illness characterized by repeated drinking of alcoholic beverages resulting in one or more of the following: (1) physiologic or psychologic dependence on alcohol; (2) impairment of physical or mental health; and (3) impairment of the individual's functioning at home, school, work, or any other sector of his life.

Of the approximately 90,000,000 persons in the United States who drink, it is estimated that about 9,000,000 are alcoholics. The damaging consequences of this widespread disorder are enormous. This disease not only affects the patient himself but more often than not it has a severe impact upon his or her immediate family, especially upon those who are psychologically and economically dependent upon the patient. Divorce rates, suicide rates, and the incidence of serious physical illness are much higher among alcoholics than in the general adult population. Excessive drinking is frequently implicated in homicides and automobile accidents.

Physicians, both generalists and specialists, encounter patients with alcoholism in all its stages: patients in whom the illness is incipient, patients who openly seek help for loss of control of their drinking, patients with physical illnesses frequently associated with alcoholism, and patients admitted to the hospital for an incidental medical or surgical illness who develop an alcohol withdrawal syndrome.

In view of its frequency and its incapacitating, sometimes fatal, consequences, it is appropriate that medical organizations such as the American Medical Association and the American College of Physicians (among others) have officially recognized alcoholism as a major health problem and have endorsed therapeutic and preventive efforts by their members. However, as Lisansky has suggested, the necessity for statements of attitudes and policies toward alcoholism probably reflects a degree of resistance or reluctance on the part of physicians to diagnose and manage alcoholism as readily as they do other disorders.[7] There are probably a number of reasons for this. Among them is the fact that the alcoholic understandably engenders hostility in others who are harmed by his drinking or who feel frustrated in their efforts to help him. One may pay lip service to alcoholism being an illness while really regarding it as willfully destructive behavior. Further, especially in relatively early or questionable cases, the physician may feel that he will anger or alienate the patient if he raises the possibility of a drinking problem or implies its possible existence by pursuing a relevant line of inquiry. The physician who has avoided learning about alcoholism and therefore feels insecure about its management may tend to avoid the diagnosis. Finally, if the physician himself drinks he may set his own drinking habits as the norm and regard drinking that is equal to or less than his own as clinically insignificant.

PHARMACOLOGY OF ETHYL ALCOHOL[1,9]

ABSORPTION

Following oral ingestion, alcohol is usually rapidly absorbed, so that measurable amounts may appear in the blood within several minutes. About 20 percent is absorbed by the stomach and the remainder in the small bowel. Complete absorption is delayed if the amount and concentration of alcohol are high enough to promote the secretion of a protective layer of mucus by the gastric mucosa and pylorospasm. Absorption is also slowed by the presence of food, particularly fatty foods, in the stomach.

DISTRIBUTION, METABOLISM, AND EXCRETION

Alcohol tends to be evenly distributed in body fluids and, of course, crosses the blood-brain and placental barriers readily. The presence of alcohol in the fetal circulation is of more than academic interest. A number of investigators have reported a pattern of malformation in infants born to severely alcoholic women which has been called the "fetal alcohol syndrome." Hanson et al estimate that the risk to the developing fetus is sufficiently high that alcoholic women should be advised and helped to avoid pregnancy until they discontinue drinking.[4]

Only about 2 to 10 percent of alcohol is excreted unchanged by the kidneys, lungs, and skin. The remainder is metabolized at a fairly steady rate which, in the average adult, is about three quarters of an ounce of whiskey per hour. This rate is relatively slightly influenced by such factors as the energy requirements of the subject and the parenteral administration of glucose and insulin. For practical purposes, the metabolic disposition of alcohol is a linear function of time. The continued ingestion of alcohol at a rate which exceeds that of metabolic disposition eventually results in intoxicating levels of alcohol concentration in blood and tissues.

The first step in the metabolism of alcohol occurs chiefly in the liver and consists in its oxidation by alcohol dehydrogenase to acetaldehyde. The latter is converted in the liver and other tissues to acetate which can be further oxidized to carbon dioxide and water. Disulfiram (Antabuse) impedes the oxidation of acetaldehyde, thus permitting the rapid accumulation of this substance to toxic levels.

During the early phase of alcohol ingestion, the period in which the blood alcohol level is rising, there is suppression of antidiuretic hormone secretion with resulting increase in urine formation. Later, however, there is a tendency to retain sodium and water. It therefore is not uncommon for an inebriated person to be in positive water balance, eventually resulting in overhydration. However, in the presence of prolonged restriction of fluid intake, vomiting, diarrhea, fever, or diaphoresis, the patient will be dehydrated. The acutely or chronically alcoholic patient therefore requires individual assessment of his state of hydration.

Alcohol appears to stimulate lipid anabolism, an effect presumably related to the development of fatty liver, which in turn may or may not be related to the development of alcoholic cirrhosis.

EFFECTS ON CNS

The principal acute physiologic effect of alcohol is upon the central nervous system, where it acts as a depressant. The apparent stimulation following alcohol ingestion results from the depression of brain stem centers which modulate cortical activity.

In most people, blood alcohol levels of 0.10 to 0.15 percent are associated with definite evidence of intoxication. Many of the early manifestations of intoxication are related to decreased inhibition demonstrated by increased talkativeness and relatively poor impulse control. A mild euphoria is sometimes succeeded by feelings of depression and anxiety, the appearance of which might be related to the effect of intoxicating levels of alcohol on neural mechanisms necessary for the normal operation of psychologic defenses. Reasoning, memory, and judgment are progressively impaired as intoxication deepens. Speech becomes rambling and slurred. Ataxia and general motor incoordination become pronounced. At blood levels of 0.30 percent or higher there is marked confusion progressing to stupor and coma as the blood level approaches 0.40 percent. The lethal concentration of blood alcohol is said to lie between 0.5 and 0.8 percent.

TOLERANCE AND DEPENDENCE

With frequently repeated or sustained use of alcohol, tolerance develops and is the result of both an increased rate of metabolic disposition and a decreased response to alcohol at receptor sites in the central nervous system. Absence of intoxication at blood alcohol levels of 0.15 percent or higher is evidence that the person has acquired a substantial tolerance to alcohol. Cross-tolerance develops to other CNS depressants such as barbiturates, other hypnotic agents, and the minor tranquilizers such as meprobamate, chlordiazepoxide, and diazepam.

Two forms of dependence, often coexisting, may develop among alcohol users. Physical dependence refers to that condition in which cessation or reduction of alcohol consumption is followed by definite physiologic changes or symptoms, ie, the withdrawal syndrome. Psychologic dependence is present when a person feels compelled to drink in order to perform certain functions in his everyday life or simply to achieve or maintain a sense of well-being.

PATTERNS OF DRINKING BEHAVIOR[5]

Not uncommonly, the alcoholic patient has a long history of normal "social" drinking which had insidiously progressed to a point at which the drinking began to pose serious problems of one kind or another in his life. It is difficult to draw a clear line which demarcates normal drinking from problem drinking or which enables the physician precisely to designate the point at which (and beyond which) "alcoholism" exists. In approaching the diagnosis of alcoholism, it is useful to bear in mind some of the characteristics of normal patterns of drinking behavior.

Some nonalcoholic drinkers tend to be quite irregular in drinking habits, accepting or offering a drink primarily on social occasions in order to promote conviviality or simply because it is customary to do so, and only very occasionally getting high or drunk. Others may establish fairly regular drinking habits, such as a drink before dinner, or a beer or two in the evening. Some may tend to drink almost exclusively on weekends, often because these are the times when social engagements are most frequent. Regardless of the pattern of drinking, however, the normal drinker retains an attitude of flexibility toward drinking, being able comfortably to forego a drink if it would interfere with other activities and being no more than mildly disappointed if he is invited to a party or dinner at which drinks are not served. If he has established a before-dinner cocktail habit, his daily consumption of whiskey is apt to be no more than three or four ounces. The normal drinker does not regularly attempt to escape from stress or painful emotion by drinking.

Problem drinking differs from normal drinking in several ways. The most obvious of these is in the excessive amount of alcoholic beverage the alcoholic drinks. He may fall into a pattern of drinking excessively every day or every weekend or once or twice a month. Although the setting of precise limits is difficult and arbitrary, most people would agree that drinking to intoxication once a month or more or becoming "high" two or more times a week constitutes habitual excessive drinking.

There are individuals who drink heavily daily but who do so in a seemingly controlled manner, not allowing their drinking to interfere with their lives in any apparent, serious way. The addiction of such persons to alcohol is revealed when circumstances, such as hospitalization, interrupt the drinking pattern and withdrawal symptoms develop.

Another pattern is episodic excessive drinking. This pattern includes the individual who drinks moderately most of the time but gets drunk several times a year. He may have a history of a progressive increase in the frequency of intoxication over a period of time. Such a history serves as a warning that the patient is heading for increasingly severe drinking problems. Another type of episodic excessive drinking is that of the alcoholic who completely abstains for weeks or months but who is inexorably drawn into a bender if he allows himself "that first drink."

In addition to the excessive amount of alcohol consumed, a striking feature of alcoholism, even in its incipient stages, is the importance that the individual attaches to drinking. This importance of drinking may take many forms: the incipient alcoholic may consider it unthinkable to eat dinner without having a drink or two first; any "occasion" whether it be one of sadness or gladness "calls for a drink"; there is keen disappointment in or actual avoidance of dinners or other social gatherings at which drinks are not served; and, finally, drinking becomes important when it becomes a source of concern to the individual who alternates between dismissing the problem and secretly feeling that drinking has somehow "gotten a grip" on him. It is almost a universal feature of early alcoholism that drinking has thus become compulsive to some degree and that the afflicted individual tends to be preoccupied or obsessed with thoughts (plans, desires, worries, regrets) about drinking.

There are several other features of pathologic patterns of drinking behavior which are of diagnostic significance. Among these is the tendency of many alcoholics to drink in order to escape from painful emotions or from the discomforts of withdrawal. This type of drinking usually draws the individual into a vicious circle. For example, the person who drinks to escape from depressive feelings sometimes finds that such feelings, after initial transient relief, actually become more intense and thus lead to more drinking. More common is the situation in which the patient experiences the "shakes," restlessness, insomnia, or other withdrawal symptoms after a few hours of relative abstinence and drinks to ameliorate discomfort; with increasing tolerance and dependence, the amount of alcohol needed to prevent or eradicate withdrawal symptoms increases. When the drinking problem has reached this stage, the alcoholic person begins to drink in the morning and intermittently throughout his waking hours in order to keep discomfort at a minimum. He may or may not drink to the point of obvious intoxication. It is extremely common for the patient, at this stage of his illness, to attempt to keep the amount of his drinking hidden from others. He sneaks drinks, hides bottles, and, when asked, will characteristically deny that he has a drinking problem and will grossly understate the amount of alcohol he consumes. The strength of the patient's addiction to alcohol is evidenced by the fact that he continues drinking in spite of the development of severe problems with health, marriage, and job that concern him and that are related to functional impairment caused by the drinking.

OTHER BEHAVIORAL ASPECTS OF ALCOHOLISM

There does not appear to be a specific personality type that is consistently associated with the development of alcoholism. Nor is there any single, specific type of social or psychologic problem which gives rise to or "underlies" this illness. In terms of personality characteristics and associated emotional problems or illness, alcoholics are a rather heterogeneous group of people. Nonetheless there are psychologic and behavioral features which seem to occur somewhat more frequently among alcoholics than in the general population. Sometimes, however, it is very difficult to determine whether particular behavioral traits and emotional problems antedated the drinking problem or are secondary to it.

As noted in the preceding section, it is extremely common for the alcoholic patient to deny that he has a drinking problem, to insist that he is not dependent upon alcohol, and grossly to understate the amount of alcohol he consumes. In addition, one is sometimes struck by the tendency of the alcoholic similarly to employ denial when dealing with other aspects of his life that would be painful for him to confront directly. With this type of patient one is tempted to speculate that the general use of denial is part of the patient's approach to life and that the drinking itself is one manifestation of the denial pattern of behavior.

Similarly, the alcoholic's use of drinking in lieu of facing his problems and actively coping with them can validly be termed self-destructive because of the dire consequences that ultimately result from such behavior. Not infrequently, the alcoholic patient also displays strikingly self-destructive behavior that is not associated with or a result of drinking. Further, drinking in lieu of actively coping with life can be viewed as passive behavior which is highly gratifying to persons with strong dependent or "oral" needs. Indeed, some alcoholic persons do appear to have strong passive-dependent needs with which they may be in severe conflict. Such individuals show a poor tolerance to frustration, tend to seek immediate gratification, and are more than usually dependent upon others for their sense of well-being.[1,6]

A substantial number of alcoholic persons have significant emotional problems which precede the full development of alcoholism or persist after sustained sobriety has been achieved. For example, the patient may have unsuccessfully struggled with feelings of inadequacy, anxiety attacks, chronic tension, or depression. Occasionally, a schizophrenic condition is more or less masked by chronic, heavy drinking.

ETIOLOGY OF ALCOHOLISM

The etiology of alcoholism is not completely understood.[8] The theories of its causation generally fall into three groups: psychologic, biochemical, and genetic. At this stage of our knowledge, these three groups of causative factors are not regarded as mutually exclusive.

We have already touched upon psychologic factors that possibly contribute to the development of alcoholism. Briefly, some alcoholics may exhibit behavioral patterns such as a propensity to use denial, self-destructiveness, strong passive-dependent needs, or all of these, which find expression in or gratification from repeated, excessive drinking. The person whose psychologic needs are frustrated because he is inhibited may resort to alcohol because of its disinhibiting effect on cerebral function. Emotionally ill persons may drink to amelioriate their suffering and ultimately become addicted to alcohol. There has long been speculation that a biochemical defect may predispose some persons to crave alcohol and to become addicted to it. Thus far no biochemical abnormality of that sort has been found.

There is evidence that in at least some alcoholics an hereditary factor is at work. Goodwin et al have reported that the incidence of alcoholism is higher among the biologic relatives of adopted alcoholics than among the adoptive relatives.[3] It also appears that the incidence of alcoholism is relatively high in some ethnic groups and low in others. However, differences in ethnic groups, races, and nations could well be related to cultural and other environmental influences.

PHYSICAL DISORDERS ASSOCIATED WITH ALCOHOLISM

The alcoholic is at risk for the development of a wide variety of physical disorders potentially affecting every system of the body. These range from simple drunkenness, resulting from the direct action of alcohol on higher nervous centers, to those which are indirectly linked to alcohol consump-

109

tion, such as the withdrawal syndromes or illnesses associated with nutritional deficiency, so common in chronic, severe alcoholism. In still other instances, the etiologic linkage between the physical illness and prolonged, excessive drinking remains uncertain. In addition, the alcoholic's life style exposes him to the risk of infections and trauma to a degree far greater than that of the general adult population.

It is beyond the scope of this book to deal with the myriad medical illnesses associated with alcoholism. We will, however, discuss the neuropsychiatric complications of this disorder.

ACUTE INTOXICATION

The clinical picture of acute intoxication does not require further elaboration. The term "pathologic intoxication" refers to (1) acute intoxication allegedly produced by small amounts of alcohol, and (2) acute intoxication in which the subject becomes temporarily psychotic, exhibiting evidence of excitement, aggressiveness, and paranoid ideation. The mental disturbance subsides as the alcohol intoxication itself takes its course. In some instances, the patient becomes stuporous and goes to sleep. Occasionally, the patient is brought to medical attention while still in a state of excitement and requires management.

BLACKOUTS

It is not rare for the chronically heavy drinker to have episodes of amnesia or "blackouts."[2,10] During these episodes, the individual may not manifest obvious behavioral abnormality or apparent memory deficit to casual observers. The amnesia appears to be predominantly anterograde. This was illustrated by the experience of a 65-year-old man with a long history of rather heavy drinking who joined his friends for cocktails and lunch prior to a football game. He drove his friends to the stadium, let them out at a convenient place, and parked the car. During the game he came to and could remember nothing that had transpired since sitting down to lunch including, much to his chagrin, where he had parked the car. Blackouts closely resemble dissociative episodes and indeed at times the observer is led to suspect a psychologic or defensive component.

WITHDRAWAL SYNDROMES

With the establishment of physiologic dependence on alcohol, withdrawal symptoms may first appear within several hours of discontinuance of alcohol consumption. Withdrawal symptoms may also occur when alcohol consumption, though continuing, has been reduced. Thus it is possible for the alcohol addict to develop withdrawal symptoms even though he has continued to drink. This phenomenon contributed to a delay in the recognition of delirium tremens as a withdrawal syndrome.

Discontinuance or marked reduction of alcohol consumption, with consequent development of withdrawal symptoms, may occur for a variety of reasons: lack of funds for purchase of alcoholic beverages, severe gastritis making alcohol consumption impossible, the advent of a medical or surgical illness necessitating hospitalization, incarceration, and, occasionally, voluntary abstinence.

TREMULOUSNESS

A relatively mild to moderate syndrome developing within a few hours of absolute or relative abstinence is extremely common. The patient exhibits a coarse tremor, made worse by purposeful movement, which may be so severe that he has difficulty holding a cup of coffee or lighting a cigarette. Tremulousness ("the shakes") is usually accompanied by varying degrees of restlessness, sweating, excessive startle reaction, and insomnia. The patient may be mildly confused and tend to misperceive the environment.

Nausea of the type which is alleviated by a drink is a common symptom and would appear to be a withdrawal symptom, as opposed to that produced by gastritis which one would expect to be aggravated by additional alcohol.

SEIZURES

During the first 24 to 48 hours of withdrawal, one or more grand mal seizures may occur. It is unusual for seizures to occur in the nonepileptic alcoholic after the first 48 hours of withdrawal.

It is important to recognize and actively treat the alcohol withdrawal syndrome while it is still early and mild or moderate in degree. Prompt intervention reduces the likelihood of the occurrence of seizures and of progression to frank delirium tremens.

ALCOHOLIC HALLUCINOSIS

Alcoholic hallucinosis refers to a condition whose onset usually occurs within one or two days of cessation of drinking and which is characterized principally by the presence of vivid auditory hallucinations in a patient with a clear sensorium. The patient hears voices which appear to come from outside himself, interprets these voices as being real, and reacts to them in accordance with their content. Although the voices may at times be neutral or even pleasant they are generally reproachful and threatening. In the latter instance, the patient reacts to the hallucinations with intense fear. Alcoholic hallucinosis varies greatly in duration, in some cases lasting only hours, in others days or weeks. Sometimes remission is followed by relapse. Occasionally, the condition becomes chronic and, with the development of ideas of reference and paranoid delusions, the clinical picture becomes indistinguishable from paranoid schizophrenia.

DELIRIUM TREMENS

This condition usually has its onset within two to seven days following cessation or reduction of alcohol consumption in the addicted person. Delirium tremens may develop in the patient who has exhibited the early withdrawal symptoms previously described or it may develop rapidly and in the absence of preceding symptoms of withdrawal. In its severe form the following symptoms and signs are present.

1. Marked impairment of cognitive function. The patient shows evidence of confusion which may fluctuate in severity during the 24-hour cycle. Disorientation in time is usually present and the patient may be confused as to place and personal situation. Memory, concentration, and judgment are markedly impaired.
2. Hallucinations of auditory, visual, and tactile types occur. Illusions or misperceptions of environmental stimuli are common. The hallucinations and illusions are often of an extremely frightening nature.
3. Excitement. The patient with delirium tremens typically reacts with intense fear to his hallucinations and illusions and may interpret environmental happenings in a frightening, paranoid manner. He may thus become combative when others approach him or he may attempt to escape from an hallucination or an imagined threat by jumping out the window.
4. Tremulousness and other signs of hyperexcitability, such as insomnia, restlessness, and being easily startled, are regularly present.
5. Nausea, vomiting, fever, tachycardia, tachypnea, sweating, and incontinence are common. In the absence of parenteral fluid administration, severe dehydration rapidly develops.

Delirium tremens is a serious medical disorder that carries a substantial mortality rate of about 10 percent, even among hospitalized patients. Medical complications, such as pancreatitis, hepatitis, pneumonia, other infections, and the sequelae of head injury, occur frequently among patients with this disorder.

In most cases, the duration of delirium tremens is three days or less.

WERNICKE AND KORSAKOFF SYNDROMES

The syndromes described by Wernicke and Korsakoff are secondary to thiamine deficiency and are primarily associated with chronic alcoholism, though they may also be found with other disorders, such as gastrointestinal disease, which interfere with the intake or utilization of essential nutrients.

Wernicke's syndrome refers to an acute neurologic disorder characterized by (1) clouding of the sensorium varying in severity from confusion, disorientation, and lack of interest in surroundings to severe apathy and more rarely to stupor or coma; (2) abnormalities of extraocular movements which may include vertical or horizontal nystagmus, ptosis, and paralysis of eye movements such as paralysis of both external recti; (3) staggering gait; and (4) symmetric polyneuropathy affecting predominantly the legs. With the passage of time and with adequate treatment improvement occurs, especially with regard to the extraocular movement symptoms and the state of apathy and acute confusion.

As improvement in the acute (Wernicke's) syndrome continues, a persisting memory disorder is apparent in about 80 percent of the cases. Korsakoff's syndrome refers to this relatively chronic disorder characterized primarily by memory loss and polyneuropathy. The memory loss involves both recent and remote events and is anterograde as well. Some patients with severe memory loss fill in the gaps in memory with confabulations. Confabulatory responses are not seen in all patients with Korsakoff's syndrome nor are they limited to this condition.

Treatment consists of hospitalization, cessation of alcohol consumption, the administration of 50 to 100 mg thiamine per day, and a nutritious diet. With treatment, improvement in memory takes place over a period of weeks or months but may be incomplete. The response of the polyneuropathy to treatment is usually slow and incomplete.

HEPATOCEREBRAL DISEASE

Apart from hepatic stupor or coma, a relatively rare form of hepatocerebral disease occurs in patients with cirrhosis and/or portal system shunts. This chronic and largely irreversible syndrome is characterized by dementia, dysarthria, ataxia, and athetosis. Hyperammonemia is found in this condition as in hepatic coma and results from failure to metabolize ammonium drived from bacterial action on intestinal proteins. This failure may result from hepatocellular disease or from shunting of blood around the liver or both.

NEUROPSYCHIATRIC DISORDERS OF UNCERTAIN ETIOLOGY

Several disorders affecting the central nervous system have been found to be associated with chronic alcoholism.[12] Their etiology is not known.

CEREBRAL ATROPHY

Atrophy of cerebral convolutions and symmetric enlargement of the lateral and third ventricles are sometimes found on pathologic examination of alcoholic patients. In such patients there may or may not have been a history of overt impairment of higher cerebral functions.

MARCHIAFAVA – BIGNAMI DISEASE

In Marchiafava-Bignami disease there are symmetric areas of demyelination in the corpus callosum and anterior commissure. The clincal picture is variable and includes aphasia, varying degrees of dementia, seizures, bilateral spasticity, paralysis, and coma.

CEREBELLAR DEGENERATION

In cerebellar degeneration there is degeneration of the neurocellular elements of the cerebellar cortex, particularly Purkinje cells, primarily affecting the vermis. The signs of cerebellar dysfunction involve mainly the trunk and legs. Nystagmus and speech disturbances are not usually present.

PONTINE MYELINOLYSIS

There is a symmetric focus of destruction of myelinated fibers in the basis pontis. If the lesion is small there are no symptoms and its presence is discovered on postmortem examination. Larger lesions produce progressive quadriparesis, coma, and death.

DIAGNOSIS AND MANAGEMENT

In clinical practice, the patient may initially present with one or more complications of alcoholism such as delirium tremens, pancreatitis, or gastrointestinal bleeding. When this is the case, the physician obviously must first attend to the complicating illness itself, deferring definitive investigation and management of the primary disorder, alcoholism, until an appropriate moment. By the latter is meant that point at which the patient is out of immediate danger to life, has a clear sensorium, and is not so distracted by distressing symptoms that he cannot understand and be interested in his drinking behavior and associated problems. All too often, regrettably, the appropriate moment for intervention with respect to the alcoholism itself passes by without any action being taken, the patient recovering from the illness episode and returning home, there to resume his alcoholic pattern of behavior until he again becomes acutely ill.

In the following sections, we will discuss the diagnosis and management of alcoholism and certain of its neuropsychiatric complications, namely, pathologic intoxication and the withdrawal syndromes. Treatment of the Wernicke and Korsakoff syndromes with adequate diet supplemented by parenteral thiamine has already been mentioned. For further discussion of the management of these syndromes and the other neurologic disorders previously described, the reader is referred to textbooks of medicine and neurology.

ALCOHOLISM

Diagnosis   In its early stages, alcoholism poses a diagnostic challenge. There are several reasons for this. The patient himself may not recognize that he has a drinking problem or he may tend to minimize his drinking. In either event, the discovery of the disorder may depend upon the physician's careful inquiry into the patient's drinking habits when the patient is seen for some other condition or for a routine check-up. Further, as already noted, it is difficult to define alcoholism precisely, so that the diagnosis may be difficult to make with certainty in incipient or borderline cases. In inquiring about the patient's drinking behavior, it is helpful matter-of-factly to point out to the patient that such an inquiry is a routine part of the examination. If there are reasons to suspect alcoholism, such as the presence of physical stigmata often associated with heavy drinking, the physician may indicate this to the patient. As previously indicated, those drinking characteristics which are associated with alcoholism include one or more of the following: (1) habitual excessive drinking such as drinking in excess of five ounces of whiskey per day or getting intoxicated once or twice a month or more often; (2) episodic excessive drinking in which periods of relative abstinence are terminated by benders several times a year or more often; (3) preoccupation with alcohol, which may take the form of assigning to alcohol a central place in one's life or of becoming worried about one's drinking; (4) feeling compelled to drink at certain times or on certain occasions or in order to escape from or to ameliorate problems, ie, psychologic dependence; (5) secret drinking; (6) continuation of drinking despite its causing serious family or economic problems in the patient's life; (7) the development of withdrawal symptoms, ie, physiologic dependence; and (8) the presence of physical stigmata, such as skin changes or physical disease commonly associated with chronic, excessive drinking.

Diagnostic evaluation includes assessment of those factors, such as family, job, social, or economic problems, which may be a product of or contribute to the patient's drinking. Especially important in this connection is the presence of an associated emotional illness such as depression, anxiety, or, less commonly, schizophrenic illness.

In conducting the evaluation it is usually helpful to include the patient's spouse or other close relative in an interview in which the patient is present. The patient's relative may not only be able to shed light on the patient's drinking behavior and associated difficulties but may also be of considerable help in management.

Management   In managing the alcoholic patient, the physician increases his chance of success if he combines frankness with a factual, nonjudgmental approach. Further, the physician is more likely to sustain his own interest in and respect for the patient if he does not expect the improbable of himself or the patient. That is to say, alcoholism is a chronic illness and, as with any chronic illness, there may be relapses after varying periods of remission. The occurrence of a relapse does not mean that the treatment plan has been a total failure but it does mean that the patient's addiction to alcohol persists. A professional, nonjudgmental attitude on the part of the physician may help the patient who has slipped back into drinking to continue treatment instead of being driven from it by his own shame or guilt.

The specific steps taken in management depend upon the severity of the drinking problem, the patient's attitudes, the presence or absence of physical dependence, associated psychologic problems, and physical complications.

For example, if the physician feels that the patient's drinking behavior is cause for concern and may eventually lead to a state of frank alcoholism but has not yet done so, he may state this opinion simply and clearly to the patient and solicit his thoughts on the matter. Candid discussions may lead to a plan acceptable to the patient whereby he curtails and modifies his drinking pattern. Such a modification might consist of limiting himself to predinner cocktails of specified amount with strict abstinence at all other times. The individual may be strongly motivated to adhere to such a regimen if he realizes that progression to alcohol addiction would necessitate total abstinence. Follow-up visits with the patient who enters into such a plan are essential.

When the diagnosis of alcoholism is warranted this fact should be stated to the patient. It is unwise to assume that the patient appreciates the real nature of his illness even if he has clearly revealed its presence by reporting his heavy drinking to the physician. Even in such an instance, the patient may not admit to himself that his drinking problem is serious and that he is an alcoholic.

Most authorities agree that the management of alcoholism requires that the patient totally and permanently abstain from drinking alcoholic beverages of any kind. When told this the patient may react with dismay and disbelief. For this and other reasons it is often essential to put the patient in contact with someone who himself has been alcoholic and who has achieved sustained sobriety. This may be done, in many communities, in two ways. The first and oldest method is by encouraging the patient to contact a local Alcoholics Anonymous (A.A.) group and to form a working relationship with one of its members. A second method, which may supplement the A.A. approach, is referral to an alcoholism clinic. The latter has on its staff trained counselors some of whom may be former alcoholics. In the clinic setting, the patient has opportunities to participate in group sessions with patients who are at the same stage of treatment as himself as well as others who are further along.

In the initial phase of abstinence, the patient may experience withdrawal symptoms. The management of these will be discussed later. At this point, however, it is worth emphasizing that the alcoholic patient may easily transfer his dependence from alcohol to another substance, such as minor tranquilizers. While the latter are often very useful, they should be prescribed for a limited period, such as three or four weeks.

The administration of disulfiram (Antabuse) may be a useful adjunct in the management of the alcoholic patient who sincerely wants to stop drinking but who is prone to yield to an impulse to drink. Disulfiram impedes the intermediary step in alcohol metabolism in which acetaldehyde is oxidized in the tissues by the action of acetaldehyde dehydrogenase. In the presence of disulfiram, the ingestion of even a small amount of alcohol results in an uncomfortable and sometimes dangerous reaction: within 5 to 10 minutes there develops a sensation of warmth in the face, followed by reddening of the face, chest, and arms, pulsating headache, nausea, vomiting, feelings of constriction in neck and chest, hypotension, marked apprehension, weakness, dizziness, and sweating. The initial flush may be replaced by pallor and orthostatic syncope may occur.

The initial dose of disulfiram is 0.5 g per day for the first week and 0.25 to 0.5 g per day thereafter. It is advisable for the patient to establish a habit of taking the drug at the same time every day, such as each morning before breakfast. It is no longer considered necessary or advisable to give the patient a "test dose" of alcohol after he has taken the drug for a few days. It is essential that the reaction to alcohol when taken in the presence of disulfiram be fully explained to the patient and that the possible danger to life of such a reaction be understood by him. The patient should be warned to avoid alcohol in disguised form such as in cough syrups, throat gargles, shaving lotion, sauces, and alcohol massages. At least four days should elapse between the discontinuation of disulfiram and the ingestion of alcohol. Contraindications to the use of disulfiram include myocardial disease, coronary insufficiency, history of coronary occlusion, psychosis, allergy, and recent ingestion of metronidazole, paraldehyde, or alcohol.

As indicated previously, evaluation of the patient with alcoholism includes the search for problems in the patient's life which may have contributed to or resulted from his drinking. In fact, in the presence of severe, prolonged drinking, significant problems in various sectors of the patient's life practically always exist and the patient is in need of counseling either by the physician or a person trained in the counseling of alcoholic patients.

Depression or some other emotional disturbance commonly becomes manifest either during the period of active drinking or during the early phase of abstinence. When emotional illness is present active treatment of it is important and may require referral to a psychiatrist experienced in the treatment of emotionally ill, alcoholic patients.

ALCOHOL INTOXICATION

In most cases, the diagnosis of alcohol intoxication is readily made by the presence of the characteristic symptoms that are familiar to everyone in combination with a history of alcohol ingestion. A common diagnostic error occurs when it is assumed that the patient's intoxicated state is due to alcohol when the patient has also taken some other CNS depressant such as a barbiturate or paraldehyde. This error can be avoided by careful history taking from the patient and other informants and by determination of the blood levels of alcohol and other suspected substances. Another type of error is that of failing to detect the presence of disorders or trauma which are only indirectly related to the intoxicated state such as skull fracture, subdural hematoma, and pneumonia.

Simple, uncomplicated states of intoxication do not usually require treatment. There is no practical way of significantly altering the time required for metabolic disposition of alcohol. The stimulant effect of coffee may be helpful and the administration of fluids, orally or parenterally, is indicated if the patient is dehydrated. The patient should be protected from environmental extremes of temperature and should not be allowed to engage in hazardous activity such as driving a car.

In those instances in which the level of intoxication is life-threatening and the patient is in coma, adequate supportive management is necessary and is essentially the same as for grave CNS depression due to other agents such as barbiturates.

PATHOLOGIC INTOXICATION

As the term is used here, pathologic intoxication refers to psychotic states precipitated by the ingestion of alcohol. In some cases it appears that the amount of alcohol ingested was small, far less than that normally required to produce intoxication. It is often difficult, however, to ascertain the amount of alcohol consumed. Determination of blood alcohol level is useful although the level required for intoxication varies considerably.

Some patients who exhibit mild confusion and depression may simply require supportive attention for a few hours until the episode wears off. Other patients, however, may be paranoid, excited, and aggressive. Such patients are best managed in a properly equipped emergency room or acute psychiatric ward. The principles of management are those already described for the violent patient (Chap. 7).

WITHDRAWAL SYNDROMES

Ideally, all patients addicted to alcohol should be hospitalized when withdrawal is undertaken, since it is quite difficult to predict severity of the withdrawal syndrome or whether a seizure will occur. In some cases, for example, delirium tremens is preceded by one or more days of mild to moderate symptoms, and in other cases the condition has a very rapid, unheralded onset. It is recognized that routinely hospitalizing all patients for withdrawal from alcohol is not feasible in most communities. However, hospitalization should be considered mandatory for the patient who is going to undertake withdrawal if there is a history of severe reaction (delirium tremens, seizures, hallucinosis) to previous withdrawals. For the patient who has already stopped drinking and is having withdrawal symptoms, hospitalization is necessary if the patient shows evidence of one or more of the following: (1) disorientation or other signs of confusion; (2) hallucinations; (3) neuromuscular hyperexcitability such as marked tremulousness, agitation, and startle reaction; (4) dehydration; (5) fever above 101 F; (6) serious medical or neurologic illness or complications; or (7) seizures in a patient who is not epileptic.

In the event that outpatient management is elected the following measures are taken.

1. Administration of a drug in the "general sedative" or "general CNS depressant" category is useful in allaying alcohol withdrawal symptoms

and in preventing seizures or delirium tremens. A benzodiazepine may be given, such as chlordiazepoxide (Librium) 50 to 150 mg by mouth in 4 divided doses per day, or diazepam 10 to 30 mg by mouth in 4 divided doses per day. If withdrawal symptoms have already appeared, an initial dose can be given parenterally, eg, 5 to 10 mg Valium slowly intravenously followed by a one-to two-hour period of observation to determine symptomatic effect. The patient should be given a four-to five-day supply of medicine. Valium is often preferred in the management of early withdrawal because of its antiseizure action.

2. Thiamine, 200 mg, should be administered intramuscularly followed by daily oral administration.

3. The patient should be seen at least weekly and tapered withdrawal of the minor tranquilizer should begin after two to three weeks of treatment.

The use of diphenylhydantoin (Dilantin) in the treatment of withdrawal seizures (in the absence of epilepsy) is debatable since the seizures are apt to be single or consist of only a brief flurry. Dilantin probably helps those patients who have previously had seizures other than withdrawal seizures.

The presence of alcoholic hallucinosis requires hospitalization. As with all alcoholic patients an adequate diet and vitamin supplements are important. Psychiatric consultation is advisable. Patients with alcoholic hallucinosis may respond to a phenothiazine or other antipsychotic drug.

Delirium Tremens   All patients with delirium tremens should be hospitalized and may require a level of medical and nursing care comparable to that of an intensive care unit. Since most patients with advanced delirium tremens are not able to take fluids by mouth, are hyperactive, and febrile, they may be dehydrated. The incidence of complications such as pancreatitis, hepatitis, and pneumonia is high. Therefore, the management of these seriously ill patients has several objectives: (1) induction of a calm state and the prevention of self-induced injury; (2) maintenance of the calm state until the illness remits; (3) correction or prevention of dehydration and electrolyte deficiency; and (4) treatment of medical complications, if any.

The patient should be restricted to bed and will commonly require physical restraints until a calm state has been achieved. Close nursing attendance is essential.

For many years paraldehyde was the drug of choice in sedating the patient with delirium tremens. While there is no question that paraldehyde is an effective drug in the management of this disorder, chlordiazepoxide (Librium) and diazepam (Valium) appear to be more effective, lend themselves more readily to parenteral administration, and have a wider margin of safety. The objective of drug treatment is rapidly to achieve a state of calmness without causing excessive CNS depression such as deep, prolonged sleep or respiratory depression. In their illuminating study, Thompson et al[11] found that no untoward reactions occurred among their patients treated with diazepam, whereas among the 17 paraldehyde-treated patients, two patients died and two others had episodes of sudden apnea. These investigators achieved the induction of a calm state in most of their patients in less than two hours by the administration of diazepam, 10 mg intravenously initially and then 5 mg intravenously every 5 minutes until the patient was calm. The amount of diazepam required to *induce* calmness varied from 15 to 160 mg in their reported series. These authors report, however, that much larger amounts may be required. After the initial induction of calmness, the patient requires maintenance doses of diazepam, 5 to 10 mg intramuscularly at intervals of 1 to 4 hours, until remission of the illness. In their series of 17 diazepam-treated patients, the mean duration of the illness was 56 hours and an average total of 155 mg of diazepam were required to *maintain* a calm but awake state.[11]

Chlordiazepoxide, 50 to 100 mg intramuscularly or intravenously, repeated at two- to four-hour intervals as necessary, is also effective in the management of this disorder.[1] The amount of chlordiazepoxide required varies considerably but is usually in the range of 300 to 500 mg per day. Intravenous injection of chlordiazepoxide or diazepam should be done slowly: 5 mg diazepam in one minute or longer; 50 to 100 mg chlordiazepoxide in one minute or longer.

Careful monitoring and intravenous administration of fluid and electrolyte requirements are essential until the patient is calm, oriented, and taking fluids by mouth. Thiamine should be administered parenterally at the beginning of therapy. During convalescence and later, vitamin supplements should be added to the diet. The detection and management of complicating illnesses in this group cannot be overemphasized. It may also be noted that the presence of a serious medical illness such as pneumonia may be associated with a somewhat longer duration of the delirium tremens.

The cessation of agitation and hallucinations and the attainment of orientation, continence, and ability to take nourishment by mouth marks the end-point of delirium tremens. Occasionally relapse may occur after a brief period of remission.

REFERENCES

1. Chafetz MF: Alcoholism and alcoholic psychoses. In Freedman AM, Kaplan HI, Sadock BJ (eds): Comprehensive Textbook of Psychiatry, 2nd ed. Baltimore, Williams and Wilkins, 1975, Chap. 23.3
2. Goodwin DW, Crane JB, Guze SB: Alcoholic "blackouts." A review and clinical study of 100 alcoholics. Am J Psychiat 126:191, 1969

3. Goodwin DW, Schulsinger F, Hermansen L, et al: Alcohol problems in adoptees raised apart from alcoholic biological parents. Arch Gen Psychiat 28:238, 1973

4. Hanson JW, Jones KL, Smith DW: Fetal alcohol syndrome. Experience with 41 patients. JAMA 235:1458, 1976

5. Jellinek EM: The Disease Concept of Alcoholism. New Haven, College and University Press, 1960

6. Knight RP: Psychodynamics of chronic alcoholism. J Nerv Ment Dis 86:538, 1937

7. Lisansky ET: Why doctors avoid the early diagnosis of alcoholism. NY State J Med 75:1788, 1975

8. Lundberg GD: Susceptibility to dependence on alcohol. An editorial. JAMA 233:356, 1975

9. Ritchie JM: The aliphatic alcohols. In Goodman LS, Gilman A (eds): The Pharmacological Basis of Therapeutics, 4th ed. New York, Macmillan, 1970, Chap. 11

10. Tamerin JS, Weiner S, Poppen R, et al: Alcohol and memory. Amnesia and short-term memory function during experimentally induced intoxication. Am J Psychiat 127:1659, 1971

11. Thompson LW, Johnson AD, Maddrey WL, et al: Diazepam and paraldehyde for treatment of severe delirium tremens. Ann Intern Med 82:175, 1975

12. Victor M, Adams RD: Alcohol. In Wintrobe MM, Thorn GW, Adams RD, et al (eds): Harrison's Principles of Internal Medicine. New York, McGraw-Hill, 1974, Chap. 111

Chapter 10

Drug Dependence

Management
Other Types of Drug Dependence
Amphetamines
Cocaine
Cannabis
Hallucinogens
Pentazocine (Talwin)
Phencyclidine

Drug dependence is "a state arising from repeated administration of a drug on a periodic or continuous basis."[18] People who are dependent on drugs commonly take them in sufficient amount to experience some degree of intoxication and tend to place their drug taking at a higher priority than many other daily activities. The various classes of drugs are associated with characteristic physical and psychologic findings during the period of drug use and during acute abstinence. Drugs commonly implicated in drug dependence include opiates, sedative–hypnotics, amphetamines, cocaine, cannabis, and hallucinogens. We will first discuss features common to all types of drug dependence, and then consider the specific types of drug dependence.

GENERAL INFORMATION

All drug dependence involves some desire or psychologic need on the part of the drug taker to repeatedly use the substance. This in itself constitutes *psychic dependence*. The drugs causing dependence are all active in the central nervous system, generally altering mood, thought, feeling, or sensation. More specifically, it appears that those drugs most likely to cause dependence have such effects as relief of tension or anxiety, production of sleep, production of elation or euphoria, alteration of sensory perception, reduction of inhibitions in social situations, and change of sexual drives and sensations.

Some classes of drugs, notably opiates and sedatives, also cause *physical dependence* when taken in large enough doses for a sufficient length of time. A person who has developed physical dependence will have a withdrawal or *abstinence* syndrome, a predictable series of physiologic changes which ensue on abrupt cessation of drug taking. The abstinence syndrome of sedative drug dependence is particularly important to recognize, as it can proceed to delirium or fatal convulsions. The development of physical dependence is accompanied by the development of *tolerance*, the same dose of drug causing a lesser effect after repeated use. Tolerance occurs by two mechanisms, a change in the rate of metabolism of the drug, and an alteration in the cellular receptor site at which the drug acts.

ETIOLOGY

There are three categories of etiologic factors in drug dependence: physiologic, psychologic, and social.

Physiologic Factors[7]   The analgesic or sedative effect of drugs, the development of tolerance, and the occurrence of an abstinence syndrome upon discontinuance of drug use are important physiologic factors. It must be stressed, however, that these alone rarely can account for the development of drug dependence, and that medically supervised use of opiate analgesics for painful acute illnesses does not lead to drug dependence. As for chronic illnesses, physicians may well decide that a patient's need for relief from severe discomfort outweighs the risks of developing dependence. In fact, studies have indicated that patients are more likely to receive too little rather than too much analgesia in usual hospital practice.

Social Factors[6]   Association with groups of drug-taking people, lack of opportunities for success, and lack of satisfying recreational outlets contribute to the development of drug dependence in many people. Family and community settings in which adults use and come to depend on such drugs as caffeine, nicotine, alcohol, or prescription medications, may influence some children to experiment with drug use. Differences in the incidence of alcoholism in English, French, Irish, and Jewish populations have been observed; reasons for these differences include family attitudes and practices in the use of alcohol.

Psychologic Factors   People who have various psychiatric disorders manifested by feelings of inadequacy, insecurity, anxiety, chronic malaise, or frank psychotic disorganization, may find such relief in the effects of some self-administered drugs that they become drug dependent.

Wikler has noted a conditioning effect; after months of documented abstinence, a former heroin user may experience the physical sensations of withdrawal and drug craving when he walks down a street where he was usually walking while begining to suffer acute abstinence, on the way to purchase his fresh supply of heroin.[19]

EFFECTS

The various classes of drugs produce distinct signs and symptoms, to be described in subsequent sections. Nonetheless, there are certain general effects common in most drug-dependent persons. Foremost is drug-seeking behavior; this often takes precedence over any other activity. The alcoholic may take a drink the first thing in the morning; the heroin user may spend rent or grocery money on heroin. Preoccupation with drug taking, as well as mind-altering effects of the drugs taken, commonly result in impairment in social functioning. The drug-dependent person may not be able to fulfill responsibilities at work or at home. The tension and anxiety from this impairment may be added to the anxiety associated with the psychologic problems which originally led to the drug use; a vicious circle is thus established.

DIAGNOSIS

Making the diagnosis of drug dependence is, of course, the first step in treatment planning. The primary physician is often in an excellent position to find the early signs of the drug dependence. Patients may either come for care of some aspect of or result of their drug taking, or they may present with other illnesses and the physician will diagnose drug dependence as a related or complicating condition.[15] To maintain an appropriate level of curiosity and suspicion, yet to avoid becoming a policeman or inquisitor, is a difficult but necessary accomplishment.

The physician should be alert to patients who come requesting specific remedies, especially sedatives or strong analgesics; he should keep careful records of prescriptions to prevent premature refilling. Patients who have recently consulted a number of other physicians, or who are taking a variety of previously prescribed drugs from several sources, may be drug-dependent persons looking for a new supply of medications, or they may have genuinely difficult medical conditions which have not responded to treatment. A few patients may present with simulated conditions in an attempt to obtain analgesics; the patient who claims to have intractable pain of uncertain origin may be wanting drugs. In other instances, the drug-dependent patient may present with minimal intoxication.

MANAGEMENT

A matter-of-fact, nonjudgmental approach to the patient is essential. He or she needs treatment, and needs sound information on the risks of continuing drug dependence. Only by establishing a professional physician–patient relationship, showing concern for the patient's condition, and gathering a thorough medical history, can the physician keep the drug-dependent patient under his care and offer definitive treatment either directly or by referral.

OPIATE DEPENDENCE

The most notorious but not the most common type of drug dependence is to the opiate class of drugs. Opiate dependence is an important condition because of the personal and family anguish, the medical complications associated with heroin use, and the social and economic effects of drug traffic in the community.

Opiates and other synthetic analgesics which can cause opiate-type drug dependence include morphine, heroin (diacetylmorphine), Dilaudid, codeine, opium (a mixture including morphine and codeine), meperidine, methadone, dextropropoxyphene, and diphenoxylate (Lomotil). The latter two are listed here because they can produce mild but definite opiate dependence syndromes. All of these medications have a combination of inhibitory and excitant effects on the central nervous system. Important pharmacologic properties that contribute to the development of opiate dependence include antianxiety effects, the development of tolerance, and the development of physical dependence.

ETIOLOGY

Pharmacologic Factors   Intravenous injection of heroin or morphine produces sensations commonly described by users as pleasurable. First, they experience a "rush" or "flush" of explosive intensity, often compared with sexual orgasm. This is followed by a more gradual feeling of warmth and relaxation pervading the body, with a sense of tranquility. The pleasurable aspects of these sensations are sufficient to offset the experience of nausea and vomiting accompanying the first several experiences with intravenous opiates.

After tolerance develops (and it develops rapidly to the analgesic and antianxiety effects of opiates) the major factor responsible for drug dependence is physical dependence, ie, the drug taker's desire to avoid the discomforts of the abstinence syndrome.

Psychologic Factors   There is no single psychiatric illness which is strongly associated with the production of opiate dependence. It does appear that many urban heroin users have suffered childhood deprivation that makes them vulnerable to emotional stresses and losses. Anxiety or

127

any kind of dysphoria may lead the drug user to seek relief by continuing drug taking. Immaturity and inability to tolerate frustration or to delay gratification are other psychologic traits found in many opiate-dependent persons.

Social Factors   Association with other users of heroin is an important determinant of urban patterns of opiate dependence. Membership in or contact with a group who use heroin generally provides the introduction to this pattern. Curiosity or thrill-seeking is the commonest explanation for starting drug use offered in medical and psychiatric histories given by these people.

The small group of people who have medically related opiate dependence have generally suffered from a combination of chronic pain and anxiety and apprehension which are related to issues beyond the simple worries directly associated with their illnesses. The psychologic factors are thought to include low self-esteem, depression, and some immaturity. Such patients can often be helped by combined, coordinated medical and psychiatric care.

RECOGNITION OF THE PATIENT

A patient may volunteer the fact of his drug dependence in giving medical history, or the physician may have to inquire diligently before finding this out. Some variables in the patient which may increase the physician's index of suspicion include presenting conditions such as serum hepatitis, subacute bacterial endocarditis, or acute respiratory depression. Also, the patient's social background, including who his friends and visitors are and how they behave, may contribute to making the diagnosis. On physical examination, the findings of needle punctures, scarring and darkening over veins, and possible skin abcesses are common in users of illicit narcotics.

The appearance of the opiate abstinence syndrome is a confirmatory phenomenon. This may occur naturally, in the patient who is away from his customary supply of drug, or the physician may elect to attempt to precipitate the abstinence syndrome by administering a narcotic antagonist. After obtaining the patient's consent, one can give 0.1 mg naloxone intravenously and observe for appearance of the acute abstinence syndrome.

Intoxication   Acute intoxication with a usual dose of an opiate causes the patient to have constricted pupils, lowered respiratory rate, and spasm of smooth muscle sphincters. The duration of these effects depends on the drug used, route of administration, and existence of tolerance. Psychic effects seem quite dependent upon the person's expectations and the setting of drug taking. The person in acute pain who receives morphine in hospital experiences relief of pain, with possible mild euphoria. Conversely, the person who injects an unknown but very small amount of heroin into himself, believing it to be a potent solution, obtains what he expects, namely, the "rush" followed by relaxation, although after tolerance develops the occurrence of euphoria per se is minimal.

Abstinence   Severity and duration of the opiate abstinence syndrome vary according to the amount, frequency, and duration of drug intake, and according to the substance used. The syndrome following abrupt cessation of morphine or heroin use, after at least three weeks of daily use, is the prototypical opiate abstinence syndrome. About 16 hours after the last dose, the patient begins to have rhinorrhea, goose flesh, lacrimation, sweating, and yawning; these increase in severity over the next several hours. Sluggish pupillary response to light is an important objective finding. Next, restlessness, insomnia, and muscular twitching and cramping develop, and the patient experiences hot and cold flashes and abdominal cramping. By the end of 36 hours of abstinence, nausea, vomiting, and diarrhea generally have developed. The peak intensity of symptoms is at 48 to 72 hours after withdrawal, and within seven to ten days all objective signs of abstinence have declined; patients may still complain of malaise, restlessness, and weakness for several weeks.

The important feature of this abstinence syndrome is that, while causing genuine discomfort, it is not life-threatening. Only a severely debilitated patient suffering from some condition such as chronic cardiac or pulmonary disease might have medical difficulty during untreated withdrawal.

MANAGEMENT

Acute opiate withdrawal can be treated best with substitution of methadone given orally and slowly reduced. When the patient exhibits rhinorrhea, goose flesh, and slow pupillary responses to light, the physician can begin treatment by prescribing 10 mg of oral methadone, to be repeated when the patient next has the objective signs of beginning withdrawal. This therapy is, of course, best carried out in an inpatient hospital setting, so control can be maintained over the patient's access to other drugs.

The patient who has been taking an average amount of heroin in most American cities will be maintained without signs of withdrawal on 30 to 40 mg of methadone daily. This dose can be reduced over one to three weeks to zero. Although oral methadone treats the abstinence syndrome, it produces little or no euphoria, especially when given under medical supervision, since it is given orally, and since tolerance to euphoric effects has already developed. Accomplishing withdrawal with a reasonable minimum of discomfort may be the first step in the opiate-dependent person's gaining enough trust in the people treating him to continue in longer-term rehabilitation. Detoxification or withdrawal alone is not enough to cause most patients to stop using opiates.[16] Follow-up care for six months to several years is necessary, and many patients may only accept this if some administrative pressures are placed on them. For example, a detoxification program can decline to accept people for repeated courses of detoxification if they do not continue with rehabilitation programs after the acute detoxification.

A wide range of services is necessary to provide treatment programs for opiate-dependent persons. Each person may have a different background and a different current situation, so the elements of a treatment plan must be chosen to meet individual needs. Psychotherapy, family therapy, educational and vocational services, legal aid, ongoing medical care, and social services including possible provision of housing or income support are all components of a complete treatment program. The staff in a program need to know enough about the behavior of drug users in general, and especially about those they are treating, to stay ahead of the client's attempts to avoid surveillance or abstinence. Urine checks to determine evidence of unauthorized drug use, and ongoing evaluation of the program to monitor the objective results with patients (employment, participation in family), are necessary to ensure the establishment of effective treatment programs.

The newer treatment approaches for opiate users are the methadone maintenance techniques, and drug-free therapeutic communities such as Synanon or Daytop Village. Methadone maintenance appears to be helpful for the person who has adopted heroin use as a life career, and who can benefit from additional vocational training and the rewards of placement in a steady job. Patients are given 40 to 120 mg methadone daily, which prevents them from getting any acute subjective pleasurable sensation if they should take an intravenous dose of heroin. Getting no "kick" from heroin, and being protected from withdrawal symptoms by methadone, they may discontinue seeking and using heroin. As part of a program providing counseling, training, and social services, methadone maintenance has been a help for many heroin users who had not been successfully treated in other programs.[5]

LAAM, L-alpha-acetylmethadol, is longer-acting than methadone; it can be administered three times weekly, in contrast to the requirement of daily doses of methadone. Nonetheless, even if patients do not receive medication daily, their visits to the maintenance clinic provide psychologic support that can often be critical in successful recovery.[11]

Communities of former heroin users, with strict enforcement of a complicated comprehensive set of social rules, provide a new total life career for the person who enters and stays. Members begin by a long and demanding application procedure, often having to appear for appointments several days in a row before being accepted. They then are assigned to menial tasks in the house, and gradually may work their way up to positions of some responsibility. Programs in public speaking, education, and peer-group therapy are the usual added components of treatment. Many people drop out early in treatment, and reliable statistics are not published. It does appear that a few persons who stay on in the program find a new kind of involvement and do not return to drug use.[13]

Studies to determine which kind of treatment program is more effective for different types of drug-dependent people have been instituted, but no definitive results are yet reported. A typology of drug users, and a matching typology of treatment approaches, would be a significant advance in our knowledge. To date, it is clear that any treatment program which leads to recovery for opiate-dependent patients involves several years of continuous outpatient care, with contact intensive enough to detect early relapse, and services comprehensive enough to provide new opportunities for those who want to change.

SEDATIVE-HYPNOTIC DEPENDENCE

While most abused opiates are obtained illegally, and alcohol is generally purchased over-the-counter, many people dependent upon sedatives can obtain their supplies by prescription. Despite the small percentage of people taking sedatives who have become dependent upon them, it has been estimated that in absolute numbers, as many as 2,000,000 Americans annually are taking more medications of the barbiturate class than is medically indicated. For these reasons, and because the withdrawal syndrome can be quite severe, the physician needs to be alert to this condition.

ETIOLOGY

All barbiturates, all potent nonbarbiturate hypnotics, with the possible exception of flurazepam, and all minor tranquilizers (including meprobamate and the benzodiazepines) can, when a person ingests them in large quantities over a period of time, cause the development of drug dependence of the sedative–hypnotic class. These medications have acute effects similar to alcohol, and the chronic effects, including drug dependence, are not dissimilar. However, sedative drug dependence is not associated with the kinds of nervous system or hepatic damage seen in alcoholism (see Chap. 9).

Development of physical dependence is a function of the variables of drug dosage and duration of continued intake. Daily doses of 400 mg of pentobarbital do not result in a state of physical dependence that leads to withdrawal convulsions or delirium. Doses above 800 mg daily, over 90 days, are highly likely to be followed by convulsions or delirium on abrupt withdrawal.[4,8] Even single hypnotic doses of glutethimide, methyprylon, or pentobarbital do cause distinct changes in REM sleep; this is a subtle but definite indication of physiologic changes which might be the earliest stage of development of physical dependence.[9]

Social and psychologic factors are the other major variables determining who may develop sedative drug dependence. People who do not tolerate anxiety or discouragement easily, and who find relief in the effects of sedatives or antianxiety medications, may well begin to use these in larger doses than their physician intends. Such people may have psychiatric syndromes of several varieties, including neuroses with much perceived anxiety; character or personality disorders with immaturity, low self-esteem, and difficulty in assertive behavior; or chronic depressions. The feature of relative passivity and inability to be assertive without being aggressive is common to many patients. In addition, the social sanction of prescription medication, ie, "if a doctor prescribed it, it must be all right," may be used by the patient to rationalize his or her increasing use of the medication.

Some patients seek the sedation or antianxiety effect of these substances, trying to escape the discomforts of emotional stress. Others may prefer the "high" which may ensue either as a paradoxical reaction after tolerance is established, or as a release of usual social–psychologic inhibitions due to the CNS-depressant effects of sedatives. Still another group use the sedatives in combination with other substances, for instance to counteract or temper the stimulant effects of amphetamines, or to self-treat the discomforts of abstinence from some other substance such as opiates or alcohol. This latter combination is particularly dangerous because the substances potentiate each other and the drug taker can unintentionally take a lethal amount.

Diazepam, even in modest doses, has been reported to lead to some dependence. Some patients experienced recurrence of anxiety and insomnia when they decreased their dose, and reacted by increasing their intake of the diazepam. Many of those who increased the dose reported that they believed they required more medication than before to obtain the same relief of symptoms. On abruptly stopping the medication, a number of patients experienced agitation, tension, insomnia, and tremulousness.[12] These symptoms resemble those of withdrawal from other sedatives. Withdrawal from larger amounts of diazepam (60 to 80 mg per day) taken over a period of several months reportedly results in a more severe syndrome which may include seizures.[14]

RECOGNITION OF THE PATIENT

The physician should consider the possibility of sedative drug dependence in patients who complain of insomnia, show no evidence of sleep

deprivation, and insist upon a specific potent medication being prescribed. Also, a patient who requests medication for anxiety or tension,
but who declines a skillful inquiry into the possible psychologic or social
sources of, and remedies for, the tension, may be more interested in the
effects of the medication than in any resolution of the underlying problems.

With the patient who has an unexpected and unexplained major seizure
or delirium, the physician should investigate whether sedative use has
been a contributing factor. A person who is known to be dependent upon
opiates should be asked if he or she is also using sedatives; this combination is not uncommon in either street heroin users or medically supplied
opiate users. Patients who report that they see several physicians currently, or who have a large supply of many medications, may well be
taking enough medications in the sedative class to have physical dependence.

Intoxication   The signs and symptoms of intoxication may also lead the
physician to inquire about sedative use. The mildest intoxication syndrome includes nystagmus on vertical gaze, slight dysarthria, and mild
ataxia or unsteadiness. With greater intake of sedatives, this may progress
to marked ataxia, drowsiness, or somnolence. In brief, the signs and
symptoms are quite similar to those of alcohol intoxication. The major
distinction is that the person using sedative medications will have none of
the medical conditions associated with alcoholism, such as liver or brain
disease.

Abstinence   Abstinence phenomena can be divided into minor, or
early, and major, or later-appearing types. The minor phenomena begin
appearing within 24 hours of abrupt withdrawal, and include apprehension, muscle weakness, tremors, postural faintness, anorexia, and
twitches. The major, serious withdrawal phenomena in sedative dependence are seizures and delirium, which develop in the second to eighth
day after withdrawal. Sleep disturbance, with less than four hours of
continuous sleep at night, is often a precursor of major withdrawal
phenomena. Paroxysmal discharges may be seen on EEG after the second
day of abstinence. These last two phenomena provide some objective
measures for diagnosis.

MANAGEMENT

When a patient is suspected of having physical dependence to sedatives,
withdrawal in a drug-free inpatient setting is the preferred treatment.
Such a patient needs the close supervision and medical and nursing care
afforded on a hospital unit, where the responsible physician can control
the amount and kind of medication the patient receives. This can be the

first step in the usually long treatment of this chronic and relapsing condition.

To determine the amount of medication necessary to safely treat the patient for withdrawal, a test dose of pentobarbital, 200 mg, should be given when there are no signs of intoxication. An hour after this dose, the patient should be examined for evidence of intoxication, looking first for nystagmus on upward gaze. A patient who is intoxicated on that first dose has no physical dependence and can be managed without further sedatives. A patient who is not intoxicated should have further doses of pentobarbital, 200 mg orally every two hours, until intoxicated. This total amount of pentobarbital necessary to reach intoxication is 100 mg over the patient's level of tolerance. Since there is cross-tolerance with all drugs of the sedative–hypnotic class, pentobarbital will substitute for any one substance or for any combination.

After finding how much pentobarbital is required to mildly intoxicate the patient, the physician can begin a schedule of medication reduction, decreasing the daily dosage by 100 mg each day. The pentobarbital should be given in four to six divided doses, to provide a steady tissue level of the medication; a bedtime dose is not necessary in addition to an evening dose. If any signs of abstinence recur, the dosage should be temporarily increased by 100 mg and the reduction continued the next day.

A patient who is already showing signs of abstinence on admission to hospital can be given the test dose then; ordinarily the test dose is given the first morning in the hospital, before breakfast.

While withdrawal is being medically managed, the longer-range treatment, including psychotherapy and rehabilitation, should be planned and instituted. As with other drug-dependence problems, only a combination of good medical management and long-range therapy, designed to offer changes in the person's abilities to cope with life problems, can lead to recovery. Often the drug use is symptomatic of personal or family difficulties which must be recognized and dealt with before the patient can give up drug dependence. In some instances the primary physician will choose to carry out the long-term therapy; for other patients he will choose consultation with and referral to a psychiatrist.

OTHER TYPES OF DRUG DEPENDENCE[1,7]

AMPHETAMINES[2]

Amphetamines, useful in treatment of narcolepsy and minimal brain damage syndromes, are misused by some people. The effects include elation and euphoria, appetite suppression, and insomnia. Although tolerance develops rather rapidly, and strong psychic dependence is a feature, little physical dependence occurs. Withdrawal is characterized by increased sleep, increased appetite, and sometimes by severe depression. For this reason, the person who suddenly stops taking large doses of amphetamines needs close supervision during withdrawal.

People who take high doses over a protracted period may develop a paranoid psychosis quite similar to acute paranoid schizophrenia. They commonly have auditory hallucinations, and may also experience tactile hallucinations or formication. This condition can be treated by hospitalization and chlorpromazine, and responds within a few days.

COCAINE[3]

Cocaine is another stimulant or activating drug, and intoxication results in euphoria and jitteriness.[3] A toxic psychosis can occur, with paranoid delusions and occasional outbursts of violence. As with amphetamines, strong psychic dependence but no physical dependence develops. Withdrawal often leads to profound but transitory depression. The toxic psychosis can be treated with antipsychotic medications. The chronic user will require psychotherapy or other specialized management.

CANNABIS

The resin of *Cannabis sativa* contains tetrahydrocannabinol, a psychoactive substance. When smoked or ingested, this results in a loss of time perception, alteration of visual and auditory perception with possible hallucinations, disorientation, and occasional tremors, ataxia, and drowsiness. Cannabis is usually taken socially, in a group, and the effects related to euphoria are dependent on the activities of the group and the person's expectations. Larger doses may result in dysphoria or depression.

No physical dependence is known to develop, but people who experience euphoria while using cannabis do often develop strong psychic dependence. Research into the possible desirable and undesirable effects of this drug is far from complete.

HALLUCINOGENS

Mescaline, derived from peyote cactus, psilocybin from several mushroom species, and some synthetic substances such as lysergic acid diethylamide (LSD) and N, N-dimethyltryptamine, can induce psychic experiences including changes in visual perceptions, hallucinations, and feelings of omnipotence. There may be a loss of contact with reality, or psychosis, but this is a variable feature depending on dosage and user expectation, as well as the social setting of drug use. Carefully planned and supervised LSD experiences have been used experimentally as part of treatment of terminally ill patients.

The patient who presents for medical care during a "bad trip" may have been taking a mixture of these substances, and physicians are properly wary of using additional medications for treatment because of problems of drug effect interaction. If an antipsychotic medication must be used, haloperidol offers the least possibility of untoward autonomic effects in the person who has taken an hallucinogen. Support, assurance, and "talking the person down," especially with friends he knows, can be helpful. If sedation is needed, diazepam, chloral hydrate, or short-acting barbiturates are useful adjuncts. Constant supervision in a quiet, well-lighted room is the mainstay of emergency treatment.

PENTAZOCINE (TALWIN)

Pentazocine, an analgesic, has opiatelike effects as well as being an opiate antagonist. Patients taking the medication for long periods develop tolerance, and a mild but definite abstinence syndrome occurs, with nervousness, insomnia, and muscle aches and pains. This can lead to further use of the medication, especially in chronically ill patients who have difficulty tolerating further discomfort. Medically supervised withdrawal is helpful in these patients, and drug dependence of this type may be prevented by judicious prescribing practices.

PHENCYCLIDINE

Phencyclidine (trade name Sernylan) is a veterinary anesthetic which can produce alterations in state of consciousness and/or psychotic symptoms in humans.[10,17] It is marketed in the street as powder, pills, and capsules, and is called PCP, angel dust, and flakes, among other names. People take it by inhaling, smoking, or ingesting it alone or in combination with other substances such as cannabis or parsley.

Acute effects include a toxic delirium, and other acute psychotic states mimicking manic or schizophrenic illnesses. Larger doses can produce seizures or coma. Chronic effects reportedly include dementia; some patients are also said to have poor impulse control, but this may antedate their use of this substance. PCP's effects on the autonomic and cerebellar areas of the nervous system give some signs which can lead to diagnosis. Patients who have taken PCP will have tachycardia with hypertension, sweating and flushing of the skin, pupillary constriction, and may have ataxia, dysarthria, and nystagmus. These signs, in combination with the psychologic changes of cognitive and emotional disorganization, should lead the physician to suspect PCP use.

Management of acute effects includes good general medical and psychiatric care. Seizures will probably respond to diazepam or barbiturates; diazepam may also be used for severe agitation. As with other "bad trips," minimal medication and the use of calm, constant companionship is the best approach.

REFERENCES

1. Brecher E: Licit and Illicit Drugs. Boston, Little, Brown, 1972
2. Cohen S: Amphetamine abuse. JAMA 231:414, 1975
3. Cohen S: Cocaine. JAMA 231:74, 1975
4. Essig C: Clinical and experimental aspects of barbiturate withdrawal convulsions. Epilepsia 8:21, 1967
5. Goldstein A: Heroin addiction and the role of methadone in its treatment. Arch Gen Psychiattry 26:291, 1972
6. Greene MH, Nightingale SL, DuPont RL: Evolving patterns of drug abuse. Ann Intern Med 83:402, 1975
7. Hofmann FG: A Handbook on Drug and Alcohol Abuse. New York, Oxford Univ Press, 1975
8. Isbell H, Altschul S, Kornetsky C, et al: Chronic barbiturate intoxication. Arch Neurol Psychiatry 64:1, 1950
9. Kales A, Preston T, Tan T-L, et al: Hypnotics and altered sleep–dream patterns. Arch Gen Psychiatry 23:211, 1970
10. Liden C, Lovejoy FH, Costello CE: Phencyclidine. Nine cases of poisoning. JAMA 234:513, 1975
11. Ling W, Charauvastra C, Kaim S, et al: Methadyl acetate and methadone as maintenance treatment for heroin addicts. Arch Gen Psychiatry 33:709, 1976
12. Maletsky BM, Klotter J: Addiction to diazepam. Int J Addict 11:95, 1976
13. Meyer R: Drug abuse rehabilitation. Curr Psychiatr Ther 14:161, 1974
14. Preskorn HS Denner LJ: Benzodiazepines and withdrawal psychosis. Report of three cases. JAMA 237:36, 1977
15. Sapira J: The narcotic addict as a medical patient. Am J Med 45:555, 1968
16. Sheffet A, Quinones M, Lavenhar MA, et al: An evaluation of detoxification as an initial step in the treatment of heroin addiction. Am J Psychiatry 133:337, 1976
17. Tong TG, Benowitz NL, Becker CE, et al: Phencyclidine poisoning. JAMA 234:512, 1975
18. World Health Organization Expert Committee on Addiction-producing Drugs: In Hofman FG: A Handbook on Drug and Alcohol Abuse. New York, Oxford Univ Press, 1975
19. Wikler A: Conditioning factors in opiate addiction and relapse. In Wilner D, Kassebaum G (eds): Narcotics. New York, McGraw-Hill, 1965

Chapter
11

Organic Brain Syndromes

Organic brain syndrome (OBS) refers to those conditions characterized by changes in mental functioning, particularly cognition, which result from diffuse or local destruction of brain tissue or from an alteration of metabolism that affects all or part of the brain. These syndromes are etiologically associated with a wide variety of disorders: trauma, intoxication, metabolic disorders, neoplasms, vascular insufficiency, infections, degenerative neurologic diseases, and occult hydrocephalus. In view of the extremely broad range of etiologic factors, diagnosis and management rest upon the physician's knowledge of general medicine and neurology. In this chapter, we will describe the mental and behavioral characteristics of the various types of OBS and some broadly applicable principles of management.

GENERAL CONSIDERATIONS

In most organic brain syndromes, the cognitive functions of the mind are the most severely affected. Cognition refers to all those mental processes involved in the acquisition and utilization of knowledge: conscious awareness, interpretation of sensory stimuli or perception, attention, concentration, memory, reasoning, and judgment. Any one or all of the components of cognition may be affected in varying degrees in OBS. Each component of cognition is functionally releated to every other component. For example, memory underlies all of the highest integrative functions of the brain. To reason; to establish orientation in time, place, or person; to decide on a goal and keep it in mind; to exercise judgment (which requires assessment of the present in the light of past experience); to speak coherently; all require the constant use of memory.

Disorders of memory are extremely common in OBS and can generally be classified into two types: anterograde amnesia and retrograde amnesia. The former refers to impairment in the ability to acquire new memories, ie, learning. Retrograde amnesia refers to difficulty in recalling information that has already been learned, ie, memories from the past. In retrograde amnesia it is common for more recently acquired information to be lost before older information is forgotten, ie, "recent memory" is usually affected more than is "remote memory." Most patients with OBS with memory impairment have a combination of anterograde and retrograde amnesia.

Affect and various aspects of behavior are also commonly affected in OBS. In fact, it is not rare for an early manifestation of organic brain disease to consist of a slowly progressive change in personality associated with emotional blunting or indifference, apathy, and inappropriate social behavior which is "out of character" for the patient. These personality changes may be extremely distressing and bewildering to the patient's family.

Finally, part of the clinical picture presented by the patient with OBS is a function of the patient's psychologic reaction to his own cerebral deficit, especially when confronted with an environmental challenge that highlights an intellectual deficit.

CLASSIFICATION OF OBS

A time-honored system of classification considers the organic brain syndromes as falling into two groups: acute brain syndrome and chronic brain syndrome. The essential difference between these two groups is that the former is reversible and the latter is irreversible. The simplicity of this classification scheme and its emphasis on the critical issue of reversibility (and hence treatability) are its major virtues. However, not all brain syndromes that have an acute mode of onset are reversible, nor are all brain syndromes that develop slowly over a long period of time irreversible. Further, this simple dichotomous scheme does not do justice to the various subtypes of organic brain syndromes.

Lipowski[6] has proposed a tentative classification of OBS which makes allowance for the diversity of syndromes encountered by the clinician. While early assessment of potential reversibility and treatability is of the greatest importance, it is nonetheless true, as Lipowski has commented, that reversibility can only be established with certainty retrospectively, that there are degrees of reversibility, and therefore the use of that one characteristic as the basis for classification is of dubious validity.

Lipowski groups organic brain syndromes as follows:

1. OBS with global cognitive impairment
2. OBS with selective psychologic deficit or abnormality
3. Symptomatic functional syndromes

The last group includes psychotic states in which there is a toxic factor and which may resemble functional emotional disorders, an example being the schizophrenialike syndrome sometimes seen with amphetamine intoxication.

OBS WITH GLOBAL COGNITIVE IMPAIRMENT

The three syndromes in this category have in common an impairment of many cognitive functions.

In delirium, a rapidly developing confusional state, the basic features of impaired cognition are typically present, namely, defective memory (retrograde and anterograde), disorientation, faulty judgment, and difficulty in concentration, comprehension, and reasoning.

Some delirious patients, though quite confused, may remain relatively quiet, inactive, and, depending upon the nature and progression of the underlying disease process, may slip into deeper levels of impaired consciousness, stupor, or coma. The EEG of this type of patient is apt to show high amplitude, slow background activity.[4]

Other delirious patients exhibit marked excitement and hyperactivity. These features are apt to be associated with visual and auditory hallucinations, often of a frightening nature, and fragmented, changing paranoid delusions. The patient may talk excitedly and in a rambling, incoherent manner.

Delirious patients, whether excited, quiet, or in between these two extremes, may pose considerable danger to themselves because of their disorientation and poor judgment. The panicky, excited, confused patient is a particular danger to himself and sometimes to others. The patient may disconnect intravenous tubing, walk off the ward, or jump out the window.

Delirious states characteristically wax and wane during the 24-hour period, tending to get worse at night. This fluctuation in the patient's condition may be fairly marked, so that if he is seen during one of his better periods (which may occur in midday) the diagnosis may be missed. If there is a history (usually from the evening nursing staff) that the patient has been irritable, unreasonable, or otherwise has exhibited periods of troublesome behavior, it is wise to suspect delirium and to examine the patient at various times in the 24-hour cycle, especially in the evening.

The causes of delirium are manifold and include drug intoxication, drug or alcohol withdrawal, head trauma, infections, vascular disease, and metabolic disorders.

SUBACUTE AMNESTIC–CONFUSIONAL STATE

Subacute amnestic –confusional state, sometimes referred to as "reversible dementia," is intermediate between delirium and dementia. The mode of onset is related to the underlying cause; the condition is apt to develop slowly and insidiously when it is etiologically associated with such conditions as slowly progressive hepatic or renal failure; hypothyroidism; chronic intoxication with barbiturates, bromides, or lead; a slowly growing intracranial neoplasm; normal pressure hydrocephalus; and so forth. The syndrome may follow an acute organic affection of the CNS such as that produced by trauma, infection, intracranial hemorrhage, cerebrovascular occlusion, and intracranial neoplasms.

The syndrome is characterized by diffuse impairment of cognitive function: patients do poorly in tasks of memory, especially of recent events, learning new facts, orientation, abstract reasoning, concentration, and comprehension. Unlike delirium, the course is usually protracted.

Of great importance is the potential, sometimes complete, reversibility of subacute amnestic –confusional states. Therefore the timely diagnosis of this syndrome is of considerable importance, since effective treatment of the underlying disorder can reverse some or all of the mental deficit and can prevent the progression to irreversible dementia.

DEMENTIA

Dementia refers to organic brain syndromes associated with cerebral cortical damage and characterized by widely varying degrees of impairment of cognitive function. The condition usually, but not always, has a slow and insidious onset. Depending upon the nature of the underlying disorder, the state of dementia may be static or progressive. Most patients with dementia, even those in whom the condition is progressive, show a considerable fluctuation in intellectual functioning, having moments of relative lucidity and periods in which cognitive functions are particularly severely impaired.

In considering etiology of the dementias it is necessary to bear in mind that the intellectual processes, which Hughlings Jackson called "the highest integrative" functions, cannot be precisely localized in the cerebral cortex. The degree of impairment of memory and other cognitive functions in the dementias is better correlated with the amount of cortex involved by the disease process than with the precise location of the lesion. Chapman and Wolff[3] reported that loss of as little as 30 g of cerebral tissue from neurosurgery could result in measurable deficits on formal psychologic testing. Patients who had lost 30 to 60 g of cerebral tissue were slowed down, tended to avoid new or challenging tasks, and fatigued easily. The same correlation between quantity of tissue lost and loss of mental capacities was observed when the former was estimated by measurement of enlarged ventricular spaces.[3]

Any process which results in substantial destruction of cortical tissue, therefore, can result in some degree of dementia; if the destructive process is progressive, the dementia also will be progressive. The dementias are thus associated with a wide variety of causative factors, including head trauma; space-occupying intracranial lesions; any condition producing sustained anoxia such as vascular narrowing or occlusion, apnea, profound shock, and carbon monoxide poisoning; CNS infections; occult hydrocephalus; and degenerative neurologic diseases. Among the latter group, the most common disorder is senile dementia. Presenile dementia or Alzheimer's disease is pathologically identical with senile dementia and is arbitrarily distinguished from it by its onset before the age of 60 years. Pick's disease is a rare form of presenile dementia which produces distinctive changes in the cortex, but is clinically indistinguishable from Alzheimer's disease.[12]

Since the demonstration of a "slow virus" infection in kuru, a dementia-producing disease affecting the natives of eastern New Guinea, three other dementias have become suspected of being the result of chronic viral infection, namely, progressive multifocal leukoencephalopathy, inclusion body encephalitis, and Creutzfeldt–Jakob disease.

Clinical Characteristics and Course   The clinical features of dementia are the result of:

1. impairment of cognitive functions
2. behavior related to disinhibition resulting from destruction of CNS centers or systems,
3. compensatory mechanisms
4. adverse psychologic reactions to the disease itself and to incidental life events.

When the disorder develops insidiously, as is typically the case with senile or presenile dementia, the initial manifestations may consist of changes in personality which may or may not be subtle. Friends and relatives note that the patient no longer seems like himself; he lacks a certain sparkle or involvement with life or concern and interest in others that he customarily possesses; perhaps his personal habits begin to deteriorate so that he is careless about dress and grooming, is late for appointments; and he does not show his usual sense of responsibility, acumen, and judgment. At first the patient's friends and relatives may react to these "personality changes" with irritation but as the patient's condition worsens they become dismayed and seek ways to obtain medical attention for the patient. In other cases, the dementia initially manifests itself not by personality changes but by memory loss, especially for recent events, which may be first noticed by the patient himself.

IMPAIRMENT OF COGNITIVE FUNCTIONS   Usually the earliest intellectual loss involves memory. Almost invariably recent memory is more severely affected than is memory for events of the remote past, but the latter too deteriorates as the disease progresses. Anterograde amnesia is present also and as this progresses the patient loses his ability to learn new facts, concepts, or skills. As retrograde and anterograde amnesia worsens, the patient cannot keep track of spatial and temporal data; he becomes disoriented, usually first in time and later in place but rarely in personal identification. Deterioration of all other intellectual faculties ensues, eg, marked impairment of abstract reasoning, inability to communicate ideas coherently, and faulty judgment.

DISINHIBITION PHENOMENA   Behavior resulting from poor control of impulses may occur early in the course of dementia or may not be observed until the disease is more advanced. It is often difficult in a particular instance to determine if a given behavior is due to lack of intact inhibitory neural systems, or if it is related to emotional blunting (lack of concern) or to grossly impaired judgment secondary to cognitive loss. It may be that all three of these factors operate together in most cases. The sorts of behavior to which we are referring are those which are inappropriate for the individual patient in the light of his particular personality and his situation in life. Thus newly acquired vulgarity of speech, uninhibited and inappropriately displayed sexual behavior, open expressions of hostility in unusual degree or fashion, spending money "foolishly," disregarding the sensitivities or needs of others, all of these and more reflect, at least in part, a markedly decreased ability to control social behavior in a manner customary and appropriate for the patient.

COMPENSATORY MECHANISMS   Patients compensate for cognitive loss in many ways. Early in the illness, the patient may openly accept his memory loss and attempt to help himself by writing things down. As the illness progresses, many patients tend to avoid situations in which the memory loss is apt to be revealed and to avoid changes and new or unfamiliar experiences. The patient's range of activities thus becomes narrowed and he becomes more isolated socially. It is not uncommon for patients with organic brain disease to be seemingly unaware of their intellectual deficits, as if they are able to deny (to some extent) the reality of their condition.

ADVERSE PSYCHOLOGIC REACTIONS   The brain-damaged patient when confronted (especially repeatedly) with an intellectual task in which he cannot succeed may lose emotional control and exhibit tantrumlike behavior. Some patients, whether at home or in the hospital, develop paranoid ideas as they become more demented. Paranoid ideas in dementia are usually fragmented and changeable rather than systematized and fixed as in paranoid schizophrenia. Hallucinations, more often auditory than visual, may occur. The demented patient's paranoia may buttress his denial of intellectual deficit, such as was the case with a forgetful older woman who accused the shopkeeper of cheating her when actually she had forgotten that she gave only a $5 bill and not a $10 one. Depression, either in reaction to the loss of intellectual function or to some other loss in the patient's life, may occur and may substantially intensify impairment of cognitive function (see Chap. 14).

OBS WITH SELECTIVE PSYCHOLOGIC DEFICIT

OBS with selective psychologic deficit is the result of focal rather than diffuse brain damage and is characterized by relatively restricted rather than global impairment of mental functioning.

AMNESTIC SYNDROMES

In amnestic syndromes memory loss is the predominant symptom. These syndromes may or may not be accompanied by unawareness of the memory loss and confabulation. In the Wernicke and Korsakoff syndromes the memory difficulty is characterized by both anterograde and retrograde amnesia; this condition, which is sometimes reversible, is associated with bilaterally symmetric lesions in the diencephalon (see Chap. 9). Anterograde amnesia, without significant retrograde amnesia, is associated with bilateral lesions of the hippocampus.[11]

HALLUCINOSIS

Hallucinosis refers to an organic brain syndrome with recurrent or persistent hallucinations in a patient with clear consciousness and no other evidence of a functional psychosis (loosened associations, mood disorder). It can be seen in alcohol withdrawal and with intoxication from drugs such as cocaine, bromides, and hallucinogens. Migraine syndromes can occasionally give this, and optic nerve or auditory nerve compression may lead to hallucinations in the respective sensory channel. A further distinction relates to the patient's insight, or belief in the reality of his hallucinatory experiences. Some patients acknowledge the hallucinations as a disease process, and therefore would not be considered psychotic. Other patients firmly believe that the hallucinations represent reality; they are by definition psychotic.

FRONTAL LOBE SYNDROMES

Frontal lobe damage probably has to be bilateral to produce the classic picture. The symptoms include poor modulation of mood with irritability, indifference, euphoria, depressionlike inactivity or apathy, loss of motivation and goal-directed behavior, poor control of impulses, and lack of initiative or spontaneity. The patient may have difficulty in maintaining attention during the interview and in abstract thinking. Recent memory may be impaired.

A basic deficit according to Oppenheimer[7] is that the patient with frontal lobe damage cannot see into the future, ie, cannot anticipate the consequences of his behavior. This concept can account for such silly behavior as that of the man who put a slice of bread smeared with jam into a toaster, and was totally surprised by the resulting mess. Similar lack of foresight may have more serious results. Oppenheimer mentions a man who decided to retrieve the cigar he had just dropped from a window; he sustained a leg fracture after jumping out to catch the cigar. He later said: "I just wanted to get it, I couldn't see what would happen to me."[7]

TEMPORAL LOBE SYNDROMES

Temporal lobe dysfunction can lead to various deficits. Bilateral amputation of temporal lobes in man or other primates results in the Klüver-Bucy syndrome with loss of appropriate fear and anger, continuous anterograde amnesia, compulsive oral behavior, and indiscriminate sexual activity.

Irritative lesions from any cause may give rise to psychomotor seizures ("temporal lobe epilepsy"). These are characterized by (1) various subjective manifestations such as feelings of depression, anxiety; distortions of perception, eg, macropsia and micropsia; depersonalization and déjà vu or jamais vu experiences; auditory and gustatory hallucinations; abdominal pain and other sensations; and (2) various motor manifestations such as repetitive activities or automatisms including lip-smacking, chewing, or engaging in some other action repeatedly; rarely there are outbursts of aggressive behavior. There is amnesia for the events of the seizure and often there is impairment of recall for events of the preictal and postictal periods.

PARIETAL LOBE SYNDROMES

Parietal lobe syndromes involve language function, with the patient unable to name objects (aphasia) or to know how to use them (apraxia) or both. A man was brought to the emergency psychiatric unit by his wife who insisted he was depressed since he was no longer able to perform as a foreman in a sheet metal works. On careful examination, it was noted that he called a hamburger a "ham sandwich." Further history indicated that the actual problem at work was that he could not tell the other men which tool to use for a particular operation, though he could show them what to do. He subsequently received irradiation for a large parietal lobe glioma, and much of his aphasia and apraxia abated.

Body image representation also requires the parietal lobes, and lesions of the nondominant parietal lobe lead to disregard of the opposite side of the body. A 57-year-old woman was admitted to psychiatric hospital for depression; in the ward she put on a sweater, leaving her left arm out of the sleeve, and denied anything was amiss when asked about it. She had a meningioma compressing her right parietal area.

ANOSOGNOSIA

Anosognosia refers to a particular type of deficit in self-representation. Denial of illness, especially denial or disregard of such neurologic conditions as hemiplegia or hemianopsia, can be extremely disturbing to family and to nursing–medical staff caring for the patient. This denial or, more properly speaking, disregard, may represent a neurologic deficit, and should be given serious attention. Anosognosia is not a localizing symptom, as the condition may result from lesions in frontal, parietal, or other areas.[13]

DEPERSONALIZATION

Depersonalization may be due to psychologic causes or may result from organic brain dysfunction. Again, it is not a localizing symptom, but may accompany epilepsy, temporal lobe disease, as well as neurotic or psychotic illnesses. The patient feels an uncanny sense that things are not quite right, not real, and that he may be a changed person or even someone else. Apparently what is lacking is a sense of participation, as if there is a failure to integrate cognitive and affective aspects of experience. Most patients who experience depersonalization describe it as strangely alien, and they retain insight in the sense that the experience is regarded as a symptom of some sort even though its origin is not understood. In schizophrenia, however, depersonalization may lead to delusional explanations of the phenomenon. Depersonalization usually is a transient or paroxysmal symptom.

SYMPTOMATIC FUNCTIONAL SYNDROMES

Symptomatic functional syndromes include psychoses which arise in the course of an organic brain disorder, improve as the organic condition resolves, and which closely resemble or are even clinically indistinguishable from schizophrenic, paranoid, and affective syndromes. There may or may not be accompanying cognitive deficits.

It is noted in Chapter 14 that an occult abdominal neoplasm such as carcinoma of the pancreas or carcinoma of the colon may be associated with severe depression; the explanation for this phenomenon is not known. It is also noted that depression can be associated with a variety of drugs such as reserpine and methyldopa. Mood alteration of a manic or depressive sort is sometimes observed with the use of cortisone, ACTH, and a variety of hallucinogenic drugs. It is not uncommon for Parkinson's disease to be associated with profound depression. More often than not, these affective states are not accompanied by the cognitive deficits which are the classic earmarks of OBS, and the toxic or other organic etiology can only be surmised by finding (1) that the history of onset of the depression or manic state is associated with toxic or organic factors and (2) that clinical remission follows removal of the organic factor. It is worth noting that drug-induced depression may be slow to remit and may require psychiatric treatment in addition to removal of the offending agent.

Schizophrenialike syndromes may be seen in association with a variety of toxic and other organic factors. Amphetamine intoxication may produce a state closely resembling paranoid schizophrenia. Viral encephalopathy,[8] lesions involving the limbic system,[9] and temporal lobe epilepsy[10] may be associated with symptom constellations that, in varying degree, resemble schizophrenic syndromes.

These organic "symptomatic functional syndromes" remind us of the critical importance of conducting careful and open-minded diagnostic evaluation of patients who present with predominantly "psychologic" symptoms.

DIAGNOSIS

In most instances the diagnosis is readily made by the presence of features characteristic of one of the types of organic brain syndromes previously described. A history of personality change or evidence of impaired cognitive function or both point to the likelihood of an organic disorder affecting cerebral function. It is possible of course to make diagnostic errors in both directions, ie, diagnosing organic affection when that is not the principal problem and vice versa. An example of the former is described in Chapter 14 where it is noted that depression, especially in the elderly, could produce a clinical picture resembling dementia. The diagnosis is usually made by obtaining a history from the patient's relatives which suggests that a depressive mood disturbance preceded impairment of cognition. The diagnosis is further supported when cognitive functions improve along with improvement of depressive symptoms with appropriate treatment. It is also possible to mistake an acute schizophrenic psychosis for delirium, although usually careful interviewing will reveal that the schizophrenic patient is not truly disoriented (though he may be delusional about people and places) and does not have memory impairment.

On the other hand, as was noted in the discussion of organically caused "symptomatic functional syndromes," it is not uncommon for mood disorders to be precipitated by toxic or other organic factors. The diagnosis is suspected by finding evidence from the history or by physical and laboratory examination of a possible organic etiology; the diagnosis subsequently is supported if symptomatic remission follows removal of the organic factor.

In any case in which OBS is diagnosed, the discernment of the precise organic etiology is obviously of critical importance. Those conditions which are partially or totally reversible with appropriate treatment must be given prime consideration in the medical and neurologic evaluation of the patient.

MANAGEMENT

The first goal of treatment is to halt or reverse the process which has given rise to the organic brain syndrome if the latter is associated with a treatable condition. It is beyond the scope of this book to review the numerous medical and surgical conditions which may cause organic brain syndromes, and which require prompt detection and specific treatment in order to arrest progression of the cerebral disorder and, in many instances, to bring about substantial or complete recovery of cerebral function. A relatively recently described condition which can simulate presenile dementia is occult hydrocephalus; some patients with this condition show remarkable return of higher cerebral function following surgical intervention.[1]

The management of delirious states associated with withdrawal from CNS depressant drugs, including alcohol, is discussed in Chapters 9 and 10. These withdrawal syndromes require the judicious use of CNS depressants with phased withdrawal over a period of time.

With the exception of OBS secondary to drug or alcohol withdrawal, it is generally prudent to keep CNS depressant medications to a minimum in managing patients with OBS. The use of barbiturates, especially in the elderly, may actually increase mental confusion and sometimes have a paradoxical effect of making agitation and restlessness worse. If a sedating or tranquilizing agent is needed, one of the benzodiazepines such as diazepam (Valium) or flurazepam (Dalmane) may be helpful, or a phenothiazine which tends to have minimal hypotensive side effect such as trifluoperazine (Stelazine) or perphenazine (Trilafon). In elderly patients and patients with OBS it is advisable to prescribe these drugs in somewhat lower dosages than those usually employed for adult patients.

It is difficult to generalize about the necessity to hospitalize the patient with OBS for diagnostic evaluation and management. It is wise to hospitalize the patient promptly under the following conditions.

1. OBS of unknown etiology, especially with recent and rapid onset
2. OBS associated with psychosis or with behavior that endangers the well-being of the patient or others
3. OBS that requires potentially hazardous diagnostic procedures, the use of which may necessitate prompt therapeutic intervention

On the other hand, insidiously developing OBS which has been present for some months or longer, especially in the elderly patient, may not require hospitalization, at least in the initial stages of evaluation and management.

The principles of management of the OBS patient have been described in the discussions of delirium tremens (Chap. 9) and the "ICU syndrome" (Chap. 5). To repeat briefly some of the salient principles of management described in those chapters, the physician provides an environment in which there is neither sensory overload nor sensory deprivation. A dull, monotonous environment can lull the patient into a nonalert state which further reduces his chance of grasping what is going on in his surroundings. The patient requires an optimum amount of stimulation and orienting cues such as wall clock, calendar, daily newspaper, and familiar people who take an interest in him, in order to enhance his ability to keep oriented in time, place, and personal situation. Too much sensory stimulation, such as excessive noise, bright lights on at all hours, complicated discussions of the treatment plan, and so forth may result in more confusion and agitation and may lead to sleep deprivation.

For the patient with dementia or other chronic brain syndrome, psychotherapy and social therapy can make a large difference in the quality of life. Support and encouragement, advice about how to limit activities appropriately, and the authoritative yet kind interest of the physician can help the patient and family adjust to many deficits. Social therapy includes golden age clubs and other organized recreation. Both mind and body should be active within feasible limits; disuse atrophy of either can bring on a worsening of the condition. The patient who has some reasons to look forward to new or interesting activities will get out of bed and begin his day with some energy. These activities are also important to the family; they cannot take full-time supervision of the patient without stress, and they must have some respite.

For managing patients with OBS, repeated examination of mental status is a valuable means of monitoring progress or deterioration. One useful instrument for doing and comparing serial mental state examination is the "mini-mental state" developed by Folstein et al.[5]

150

As some patients become progressively more feeble or confused, a nursing home may appear to offer better care than continued home care. Choosing a nursing home is a challenge for physician and family and often they will want the help of a social worker who has experience in this field. Some factors to consider in selection of a nursing home include competence of administration, levels of health care offered, location, planned activities, and association with medical facilities for more acute care if needed.[2] Patient and family both will fare better if this choice is made carefully and thoughtfully.

REFERENCES

1. Benson DF: The hydrocephalic dementias. In Benson DF, Blumer D (eds): Psychiatric Aspects of Neurologic Disease. New York, Grune & Stratton, 1975
2. Busse EW: Aging and psychiatric disorders of late life. In Arieti S (ed): American Handbook of Psychiatry, Vol. 4. New York, Basic Books, 1975
3. Chapman LF, Wolff HG: The cerebral hemispheres and the highest integrative functions of man. Arch Neurol 1:357, 1959
4. Engel GL, Romano J: Delirium, a syndrome of cerebral insufficiency. J Chronic Dis 9:260, 1959
5. Folstein MF, Folstein SE, McHugh PR: "Mini-mental state." J Psychiat Res 12:189, 1975
6. Lipowski ZJ: Organic brain syndromes. Overview and classification. In Benson DS, Blumer D (eds): Psychiatric Aspects of Neurologic Disease. New York, Grune, & Stratton, 1975
7. Oppenheimer H: Clinical Psychiatry. New York, Harper & Row, 1971
8. Penn H, Racy J, Lapham L, et al: Catatonic behavior, viral encephalopathy, and death. Arch Gen Psychiat 27:758, 1972
9. Pincus J, Tucker G: Behavioral Neurology. New York, Oxford Univ Press, 1974
10. Slater E, Beard AW, Glithero E: Schizophrenialike psychoses of epilepsy. Int J Psychiatry 1:6, 1965
11. Victor M: The amnesic syndrome and its anatomical basis. Can Med Assoc J 100:1115, 1969
12. Wells CE: Dementia reconsidered. Arch Gen Psychiat 26:385, 1972
13. Weinstein EA, Kahn RL: Denial of Illness. Springfield, Ill, Thomas, 1955

Chapter

12

Neuroses and Personality Disorders

While it is true that the management of persons with severe neuroses often requires intensive treatment that is beyond the available time, interest, and training of the nonpsychiatrist physician, it is also true that persons with these disorders often first turn to their family physician for help.

It is far less common for the individual with a personality disorder uncomplicated by any other difficulty to consult the family physician. It is not rare, however, for maladaptive patterns of behavior which characterize personality disorders to become manifest in those situations in which the patient with personality disorder seeks attention for incidental medical illness.

DEFINITIONS

NEUROSES

Neuroses are a group of syndromes characterized by some degree of anxiety, often accompanied by other symptoms such as phobias, obsessions, compulsions, conversion reactions, and hypochondriacal complaints.[2,7,8] The latter symptoms arise, at least in part, as a result of conscious and unconscious adaptive processes by which the individual attempts to avoid or reduce anxiety. Anxiety itself, in its acute form, is one of the most painful mental states to which the human being is subject. In this connection it is of interest that anxiety shares etymologic roots with anguish (Latin angere, to strangle).

The several neurotic syndromes are named in accordance with the particular symptoms that dominate the clinical picture. Thus, if the condition is characterized principally by various manifestations of acute or chronic anxiety, it is considered anxiety neurosis. If obsessions and compulsions predominate, the condition is obsessive-compulsive neurosis, and so forth.

It is not rare for neurotic patients to engage in obviously irrational behavior. When this is the case, the neurotic person, unlike a psychotic individual, is apt to recognize the irrationality of his behavior. For example, the phobic patient may avoid elevators, not because he has a delusion about them, but in order to avoid anxiety; as a rule, he himself is mystified by his particular phobia.

In this chapter we will discuss anxiety neurosis at some length, since it is a condition which commonly requires careful diagnostic evaluation and initial management by the general physician. Phobic states and obsessive-compulsive neurosis are discussed more briefly. Conversion disorders and hypochondriasis are discussed in Chapter 13 and neurotic depression in the chapter on mood disorders.

PERSONALITY DISORDERS

Personality disorders are characterized by constellations of character traits, attitudes, and patterns of behavior which are deeply ingrained,

153

usually having been present since adolescence or earlier, and which interfere, to some degree, with the individual's adaptation to life.[2,3,8] Individuals with personality disorders may have no symptoms, or only minimal ones of neurosis or other psychiatric illness. On the other hand, the person with symptoms of a neurosis often presents evidence of preexisting personality disorder.

The salient features of various personality disorders will be briefly described. Most family physicians will not be involved in the psychotherapeutic modification of attitudes and behavior patterns of their patients with these disorders. A sensitive awareness of the patient's attitudes and behavioral patterns, however, may be useful to the physician in the management of medical illnesses in persons with personality disorders.

ANXIETY NEUROSIS

Anxiety neurosis, in common with the other neuroses, usually has its onset in young adulthood. This condition is characterized by one or both of the following: acute attacks of anxiety, or chronic tension state or chronic anxiety.

ACUTE ANXIETY

In an acute attack of anxiety the patient experiences a sudden onset of symptoms, predominant among which is an emotion similar or identical to that of fear. In a severe attack the anxiety may be of such intensity that the patient describes himself as terrified or panicked. In a typical attack there are signs and symptoms of sympathetic discharge: tachycardia, palpitations, sweating, dry mouth, pupillary dilation, and blurring of vision. Transient pain over the precordium or in the upper left quadrant of the chest, not related to exertion, may occur. The patient may show a fine tremor of the hands and usually is restless. He may complain of not being able to get a deep or satisfying breath or of having a suffocating feeling while objectively exhibiting tachypnea. Hyperventilation, in turn, may lead to respiratory alkalosis resulting in paresthesia of the extremities and circumoral region, dizziness, lightheadedness, fullness in the head, or a feeling of weakness or faintness. Frank tetany with carpopedal spasm is unusual.[4]

More often than not, the patient is not consciously aware of any precipitating factor, but once the attack has begun he is apt to focus his apprehension upon something specific. This commonly takes the form of fear that the cardiac palpitations signal an impending heart attack and

154

death. The patient may fear that he is going crazy, that he will suffocate, or that something terrible which he cannot specify is about to happen to him.

The attacks may last from a few minutes to several hours. The patient may have a single attack only, an occasional sporadic attack, or a cluster of attacks over a period of several weeks or months.

CHRONIC ANXIETY

Chronic anxiety has also been referred to as Da Costa's syndrome, irritable heart, and neurocirculatory asthenia.

The patient with this disorder is chronically tense, worried, vaguely apprehensive, and sometimes irritable. The content of the apprehension may involve a variety of issues such as his own health, family, or work. The patient typically has a variety of somatic complaints, some of which appear to be secondary to sustained tension of skeletal muscles such as headaches in the occipital or bitemporal regions, backache, or aching in the posterior part of the neck. The palms may be cool and moist. The patient may show a fine tremor of the hands and mild restlessness. He may complain of uncomfortable epigastric sensations such as "butterflies in the stomach" and may occasionally have an episode of diarrhea. Difficulty in getting to sleep is quite common and he may awaken in the morning feeling tired. Chronic fatigue may be present through most of the day and its severity bears no clear relationship to exercise. The feeling of tiredness may be temporarily allayed when the patient becomes absorbed in some activity.

As noted above, the chronically anxious patient may also have an occasional attack of acute anxiety. Symptoms of chronic anxiety, once established, tend to fluctuate in severity from time to time.

DIAGNOSIS

In most instances, the diagnosis of anxiety neurosis, acute or chronic, is readily made on the basis of the characteristic features described above. It is possible, however, for anxiety neurosis to be mimicked by medical disorders. Indeed, the patient may make it clear that he himself needs to be convinced that he does not have an organic medical disease.

Hyperthyroidism may closely simulate the anxiety state and indeed may be accompanied by considerable tension and apprehension. The tachycardia of anxiety neurosis is apt to wax and wane with the occurrence and remission of spells of anxiety, as contrasted with the more constantly present tachycardia of hyperthyroidism. However, the clinical features of these two disorders can be sufficiently similar that the physician may want to rule out hyperthyroidism with appropriate laboratory tests.

Caffeinism is by no means rare and is characterized by fine tremor of the hands, irritability, tenseness, restlessness, and difficulty in getting to sleep. The diagnosis is supported by a history of drinking coffee or tea in excessive quantity and by remission of symptoms following abstinence or moderation of drinking caffeine-containing beverages.[5] A somewhat similar picture may be seen with the chronic use of other stimulants such as dextroamphetamine and methylphenidate (Ritalin). It should be kept in mind that patients with anxiety, especially chronic anxiety, may be somewhat prone to drink coffee or tea excessively or to take drugs of both the stimulant and sedative type.

Recurrent, acute attacks of anxiety must be differentiated from other disorders which are characterized by recurrent, acute episodes. Acute episodes of hypertension and tachycardia associated with pheochromocytoma must be considered. Hypoglycemic episodes from whatever cause may mimic acute spells of anxiety. Rather uncommonly, epilepsy may produce recurrent episodes of fear and symptoms associated with sympathetic discharge.

As mentioned above, acute anxiety may be sufficiently severe that the patient can be described as being in a state of panic. In addition to anxiety neurosis, panic states are also observed in association with the ingestion of hallucinogenic substances, such as LSD or mescaline. Panic states may also be observed in dextroamphetamine intoxication and in schizophrenic disorders.

In the early stages of withdrawal from CNS-depressant drugs such as the barbiturates, minor tranquilizers, and alcohol, the addicted person may display symptoms virtually indistinguishable from those of the anxiety state. The recent drug and alcohol ingestion history is thus of crucial importance in ruling out states of both intoxication and abstinence syndromes which may mimic anxiety.

MANAGEMENT

The management of patients with anxiety neurosis depends in part on the symptomatic state of the patient at the time he is seen by the physician.

In the management of an acute attack of anxiety, the physician keeps in mind that the patient probably has one or more specific fears, such as fear that he will die of a heart attack, will suffocate, or is losing his mind. The first task, therefore is to give the patient effective reassurance that will help him to realize that his fears are baseless. Effective reassurance is communicated to the acutely anxious patient in several ways:

1. Through the display of genuine interest in the patient's description of his anxiety experience.
2. By calmly proceeding to take the history, focusing on particularly relevant items such as a history of similar attacks in the past, and so forth.

3. By doing a physical examination in a calm, unhurried manner.
4. By offering the patient one's diagnostic impression that he is having acute anxiety; this diagnostic impression may or may not be qualified by telling the patient that one wishes to do certain further tests or examinations to be certain of the diagnosis.
5. By offering the patient a clear, simple explanation of what an acute attack of anxiety is, including the symptoms associated with the release of epinephrine that occurs with sympatheticoadrenal discharge.

The basic idea of all this is to establish a relationship of confidence and trust, and within the context of such a relationship to offer the patient an explanation, in terms he can understand, of his present condition, ie, to give the patient an opportunity to attain a measure of cognitive mastery of the anxiety experience. The patient needs to be reassured that while anxiety attacks are indeed frightening they do not cause heart attacks, sudden death, insanity, or whatever the patient's specific fear happens to be.

In our opinion, it is preferable to manage the acute anxiety attack by means of a psychotherapeutic approach such as that described above, without recourse to an antianxiety drug. If, however, the physician decides a medication is necessary, the best choice is an oral preparation such as diazepam (Valium) 10 mg, rather than a parenteral one. The patient can easily use the tablets to help control future attacks of anxiety. The patient who has recurrent anxiety attacks should be actively encouraged to recall the physician's description of the physiology of anxiety and his assurance that acute anxiety will not cause the patient's fears of medical catastrophe to be realized.

The basic principles of management, as outlined above, also hold for the patient with chronic anxiety, the difference being that the chronically anxious patient's need for effective reassurance is not so immediately pressing or dramatic. The effectiveness of the physician's reassurance may hinge in good part on the patient's being convinced that the physician is conducting a thorough examination and is being open and candid with him as the medical evaluation proceeds.

The recurrently or chronically anxious patient should be encouraged to make observations about himself and his everyday experiences in order to see if he can detect some correlation between life events or reactions to events and the waxing or waning of his symptoms. Such perception on the part of the patient will not only afford him increased opportunity to discuss anxiety-provoking experiences or concerns with others, including the physician, but may also have the effect of making his anxiety symptoms seem less mysterious and foreign. Further, such an approach will help the patient to accept referral to a psychotherapist when, in the physician's judgment, such a referral is indicated. The physician should consider referral for psychotherapy when the patient's symptoms persist or persistently recur beyond a few weeks in spite of the physician's supportive treatment.

The above approach to the chronically anxious patient may be supplemented, when necessary, with the administration of antianxiety drugs such as diazepam or chlordiazepoxide (Librium). It is advisable to prescribe such agents for specified periods of time, such as four weeks, rather than on an open-ended basis. During the specified time period, the patient may be instructed to take up to a specific daily amount on an as-needed basis. These drugs, while useful in reducing anxiety, do not appear to be effective in preventing attacks of acute anxiety. The antianxiety drugs are further discussed in Chapter 18.

PHOBIC NEUROSIS

In phobic neurosis the patient has a fear of an object or situation even though he recognizes that the feared object or situation does not pose a realistic threat to him.[1] Common examples are fear of heights (acrophobia), fear of going out in open areas alone (agoraphobia), and fear of closed places (claustrophobia). The not uncommon fear of airplane travel may combine elements of fear of an enclosed place, heights, and fear of falling or crashing. The phobic patient naturally avoids the feared object or situation and, when deliberately or inadvertently exposed to it, experiences severe anxiety. A frequent accompaniment of the fear of going out or traveling alone is fear of fainting or of becoming ill in a situation when there will be no one to take care of the patient.

Occasionally the origin of the phobia is directly traceable to a conditioning experience. Probably the most common example of this is afforded by the patient who reports that his phobia began when he had an acute attack of anxiety in a certain situation, such as while driving a car, and that since that experience he has been afraid to drive a car lest the dreadful experience (anxiety) recur. On the one hand, such a patient has developed a fear of fear. On the other hand, he now has the feeling of being able to avoid anxiety by avoiding a specific situation, ie, a feeling of having control over a sudden attack of anxiety that strikes with no apparent warning. It can thus be seen that the phobia has a certain psychologic value for the patient.

Less commonly, the phobic patient has a history of some other kind of conditioning experience that initiated the phobia, such as a fear of animals following a frightening experience with a specific animal.

It is typical for the phobia, once established, to spread beyond its original circumstances, eg, from fear of traveling by car alone to fear of any mode of travel alone. Further, the avoidance of the feared situation serves to intensify the patient's dread of it.

More often than not, the patient cannot recall a conditioning experience from which the onset of the phobic neurosis can be dated. Psychiatric theories hold that in such instances the phobic object or situation is the symbolic representation of an unconscious, anxiety-laden conflict.

DIAGNOSIS AND MANAGEMENT

Diagnosis does not usually present a problem. However, it should be remembered that like any neurotic symptom, phobias can occur in the course of schizophrenic illness. Occasionally, the fearfulness of depressed patients may bear some resemblance to phobic neurosis. It is not uncommon for the person whose life has been severely restricted and impoverished by a phobic neurosis to become secondarily depressed.

It is advisable to refer the patient with a phobic neurosis producing significant disability for psychiatric treatment, which may consist of supportive therapy with encouragement gradually to confront the feared object or situation, a more systematic behavioral therapy such as desensitization, psychoanalytic psychotherapy, or some combination of these. The judicious use of antianxiety drugs may usefully supplement psychotherapy.

OBSESSIVE-COMPULSIVE NEUROSIS

Obsession refers to the persistent intrusion into consciousness of thoughts or urges which are unwanted and which are usually regarded by the patient as alien or contrary to his consciously held values, morals, or sense of propriety.[8] Obsessive thoughts may have a wide variety of content such as blasphemous ideas or ideas concerning horrible accidents, disease, mutilation, or death involving strangers, friends, or loved ones. Sometimes the recurring thought is that of a frightening urge to do harm to someone in which case fear (and avoidance) of potential weapons, such as knives, may develop. The obsession may be concerned with dirt and bacteria, the patient being fearful of contaminating others or being contaminated by others or both.

While the obsessive-compulsive patient knows that his obsessive thoughts cannot in fact do anyone any harm, he nonetheless feels compelled to engage in certain compulsive rituals in order to protect others from harm or to undo the harm which his thoughts may have caused. In spite of the patient's conscious disclaimer of the power of his thoughts, it is as though part of his mind believes in the magic power of his thoughts and equally believes in the magic power of his compulsive rituals to protect others from harm. Compulsion rituals may consist in handwashing, counting, long prayers, and rigidly adhering to numerous regulations of everyday routines. In severe cases, the patient's waking life may be largely consumed by an endless series of obsessions and compulsions in which event his suffering is extreme.

In mild and transient form, this neurosis is probably quite widespread. Indeed it is likely that everyone is occasionally afflicted with a mild obsession, such as being haunted by doubts about turning off the stove even though one "almost" knows that he turned it off. In severe form, obsessive-compulsive neurosis is relatively uncommon.

DIAGNOSIS AND MANAGEMENT

When present in severe degree the diagnosis is apparent from the patient's own description of his tormenting condition. It should be kept in mind, however, that the development of an obsessive-compulsive state can be seen in the early stages of schizophrenic illness and during recovery from that disorder. In addition, it is not rare for the patient with obsessive-compulsive neurosis to become depressed.

It is advisable to refer the patient with this disorder to a psychiatrist for further evaluation and treatment.

PERSONALITY DISORDERS

Personality or character refers to the relatively enduring or permanent traits, attitudes, and patterns of behavior which typify an individual. Generally speaking it is necessary to have experiences with a person over a period of time and in varying circumstances before one is able to speak with confidence of his character, and even then there are ample opportunities for misjudgment. Eventually though, in the course of a prolonged or intensive relationship, one can decide that a given individual is relatively conscientious, meticulous, careful, deliberate, honest, flexible, reliable, or is relatively uncaring, sloppy, careless, impulsive, dishonest, rigid, unreliable, and so forth. One may also make observations that do not so clearly reflect value judgments, such as noting that a person is quiet, outgoing, sober, cheerful, liberal, or conservative. It is obvious that some of these traits and many others tend to occur together or cluster. In spite of this, however, there is no satisfactory scheme for classifying normal personalities. To some extent, this also holds true for personality disorders.

Personality disorders are characterized by constellations of character traits, attitudes, and patterns of behavior which interfere, to some degree, with the individual's adaptation to life.[2,3] The characteristic features of personality disorders are deeply ingrained, having been present in adolescence or earlier, and are difficult to modify. The diagnosis of a personality disorder *alone* implies that at the time of the diagnostic evaluation, symptoms indicative of other psychiatric disorders, such as a neurosis, are minimal or absent. However, it is not unusual for the physician to discern the presence of a personality disorder in a patient who has developed symptoms of neurosis or some other illness.

CLASSIFICATION AND DIAGNOSIS

The basis for diagnostic classification of personality disorders is similar to that of the neuroses in that the diagnosis is determined by those features which are predominant.[2] In practice, however, it is not uncommon to find that individuals do not fit neatly into any of these categories, sometimes exhibiting character traits of more than one type of personality disorder or traits that do not clearly belong to any of the types in the classification scheme.

Some of the more common personality disorders and their distinguishing features are listed in Table 1. It will be noted that many of the manifestations of character disorders are present in minor form in healthy personalities. Therefore, the diagnosis of personality disorder requires that these features be somewhat pronounced and associated with impairment of adaptation. Under conditions of stress or with organic brain damage, features of personality disorder often become accentuated.

Personality disorders generally do not appear to be on a continuum with neurotic or psychotic illness. Most individuals with schizoid personality do not eventually become afflicted with schizophrenic illness and not all schizophrenic patients have a preillness history of schizoid personality. When a patient with a given personality disorder decompensates the resulting neurotic or psychotic illness may or may not appear to involve an accentuation of the preexisting personality. For example, an obsessive-compulsive person who becomes ill may develop an obsessive-compulsive neurosis, or a depression, or, more rarely, a schizophrenic illness.

MANAGEMENT

The patient with personality disorder of serious degree should be referred to the psychiatrist for evaluation, even though psychiatric treatment of some character disorders (such as antisocial personality) may not be effective.[3] The best response to psychiatric treatment occurs in those individuals who are capable of feeling anxiety and guilt, and who have become uncomfortable or dissatisfied with their own maladaptive patterns of behavior.

Antisocial persons may seek medical help for incidental illness or for

Table 1. Personality Disorders

PERSONALITY DISORDER TYPE	SALIENT FEATURES
1. Antisocial personality	Has history of poor adjustment in school: academic failure, truancy, frequent arguments and fights; poor job performance: undependable, quitting without notice, getting fired; frequent conflicts with the law: larceny, robbery, rape, etc; social behavior dominated by hedonism, poor impulse control, lying, charming or "conning" people, defective sense of guilt, shallow relationships, and failure to learn from experience
2. Asthenic personality	Tires easily, is low in energy and enthusiasm, overly sensitive to physical or emotional stress
3. Cyclothymic personality	Has mood swings of depression, elation, or both, which are of moderate degree and short duration, usually occurring without apparent precipitating factors
4. Explosive personality	Tends to react with intense emotion, such as rage, to relatively minor provocation; temper outbursts are often followed by remorse
5. Hysterical (histrionic) personality	Tends to be excitable, histrionic, self-centered, attention-seeking, and seductive
6. Inadequate personality	Tends to be inept and ineffective, has poor judgment, frequently fails socially and at work, in spite of average educational opportunity and intelligence as measured by psychologic tests
7. Obsessive-compulsive personality	Tends to be unusually conscientious, dutiful, perfectionistic, inhibited; is often ambivalent and tends to doubt his own opinions and decisions
8. Paranoid personality	Shows behavior characterized by tendency to be rigid, opinionated, jealous, resentful, suspicious; is quick to blame others for his problems
9. Passive–aggressive personality	Tends to express aggression passively by procrastination, pouting, stubborn withholding, and obstructionism
10. Passive–dependent personality	Tends to lack self-confidence; often feels indecisive and clings to others for guidance, reassurance, and support
11. Schizoid personality	Feels vulnerable and therefore avoids close or competitive relationships; tends to be seclusive, aloof, does not display feelings readily, daydreams

From Harvey AM, Johns RJ, Owens AH, Ross RS (eds): The Principles and Practice of Medicine, 19th ed. New York, Appleton, 1976 medical complications associated with their antisocial behavior. Alcohol or drug misuse with associated organic complications, venereal disease, and physical trauma from fights and accidents may cause the antisocial person to have a genuine need for medical help. However, he may also contact the physician in the guise of seeking medical help, while actually intending to use the physician or the hospital for some other purpose, such as obtaining drugs or evading legal prosecution. The recognition of antisocial personality is important so that the physician can avoid being manipulated (which helps neither the patient nor the doctor), while at the same time offering needed medical help for any somatic illness that may be present. The physician may refer the patient to a psychiatrist for evaluation but the patient may not cooperate with the referral if he sees no immediate gain for himself.[10]

We have noted in Chapters 3, 4, and 5 that personality type is correlated with the way patients feel and behave when they become physically ill and that, as a corollary, the physician tailors his approach to management in accordance with the personality of the patient. For example, in dealing with a paranoid personality the physician is careful to communicate clearly, to avoid ambiguities, to invite the patient to ask questions, and to avoid bedside staff conferences in which the conversation is sprinkled with mysterious medical terms.

TRANSIENT SITUATIONAL DISTURBANCES

Transient situational disturbances refer to emotional states such as fear, grief, depression, and irritability, which occur as a reaction to severe environmental stress in persons in whom there is no evidence of underlying mental disorder.[2,6,9] Symptoms recede as the stress diminishes. For example, a conscientious person with heavy responsibilities may react with considerable apprehension and despondency to being laid off from work particularly at a time when jobs are scarce. Finding work restores his sense of well-being. If such a distraught individual were seen during a period of unemployment, his condition would be considered an adjustment reaction of adult life.

REFERENCES

1. Agras S, Chapin HN, Oliveau DC: The natural history of phobia, course and prognosis. Arch Gen Psychiatry 26:315, 1972
2. American Psychiatric Association: Diagnostic and Statistical Manual of Mental Disorders, 2nd ed. Washington, DC, APA, 1968
3. Cleckley H: The Mask of Sanity. St Louis, Mosby, 1976

4. Engel GL, Ferris EB, Logan M: Hyperventilation. Analysis of clinical symptomatology. Ann Intern Med 27:683, 1947
5. Greden JE: Anxiety or caffeinism: Diagnostic dilemma. Am J Psychiatry 131:1089, 1974
6. Horowitz M: Stress response syndromes. Arch Gen Psychiatry 31:768, 1974
7. Nemiah JC: Neuroses. In Freedman AM, Kaplan, HI, Sadock BJ (eds): Comprehensive Textbook of Psychiatry, 2nd ed. Baltimore, Williams and Wilkins, 1975, Chap 21
8. Shapiro D: Neurotic Styles. New York, Basic Books 1965
9. Vaillant GE: Theoretical hierarchy of adaptive ego mechanisms. Arch Gen Psychiatry 24:107, 1971
10. Vaillant GE: Sociopathy as a human process. Arch Gen Psychiatry 32:178, 1975

Chapter

13

Conversion Disorders and Hypochondriasis

DEFINITIONS

CONVERSION DISORDER

Conversion disorder refers to any condition characterized by physical symptoms denoting loss or disorder of a bodily function for which no evidence of an organic basis is discernible and for which examination does reveal evidence to support psychogenic etiology. Conversion symptoms involve those functions subserved by the somatosensory nervous system and the special senses and include blindness, deafness, paresthesias, anesthesia, pain, tremor, weakness, paralysis, and seizurelike episodes.

Psychophysiologic symptoms are distinguished from conversion symptoms by the fact that the former are the result of physiologic changes which in turn are the consequences of psychologic reactions. For example, the occipital pain of tension headache results from sustained contraction of skeletal muscles in the occipitonuchal region; therefore the occipital pain itself is the result of a physiologic process and is not a conversion symptom.

Since psychophysiologic and conversion symptoms occur in patients with a wide variety of emotional disturbances, it is not surprising that both may occur in the same patient, either simultaneously or at different times. Briquet's syndrome or conversion hysteria refers to a chronic or recurrent neurotic condition characterized primarily by a marked tendency repeatedly to develop a variety of conversion and psychophysiologic symptoms.[4,5]

HYPOCHONDRIASIS

Hypochondriasis refers to a condition in which the patient tends to be preoccupied with bodily functions and to be constantly worried about his physical health. Unlike conversion disorder, however, there is no loss or disorder of bodily function.

CONVERSION DISORDERS

A CONCEPTUAL MODEL[2,3,6,7]

Freud originally coined the term conversion to refer to a process which resulted from an unconscious conflict brought about by the mobilization of a wish or fantasy which is repressed because its sexual content is not acceptable to the patient's conscious mind; he theorized that the libidinal energy attached to the "unbearable idea" was discharged by being transmuted or converted into a physical symptom. This theoretical concept has been seriously challenged as indeed has been the libido theory itself. Many students of human behavior assert that while neurotic conflicts often involve sexual issues they do not invariably do so.

Even if one rejects the original Freudian formulation, conversion remains very useful as a metaphoric term that denotes a psychologic process in which the patient defends himself against unbearably painful feelings by developing physical symptoms. That is, it is as though the patient has unconsciously "converted" a psychologic problem into a physical one. According to this concept, the physical symptoms, unpleasant though they may be, serve partially to replace and to distract the patient from painful emotions. For example, if the emotional problem is one about which the patient feels hopeless he may, in developing a conversion symptom, have substituted for it a problem for which he has hope that medical treatment will be effective. Further, the patient with a conversion symptom is in the relatively passive role of seeking medication or surgery, as opposed to the more active one of facing and resolving the underlying problem. Apparent physical sickness also brings with it socially approved gratification of needs to be dependent and to be the object of sympathetic concern.

It is to be stressed that the patient with conversion symptoms, in contrast to the malingerer, experiences his symptoms as quite real. This was exemplified by the patient described in Chapter 7 who had conversion anesthesia and underwent tracheostomy without apparent discomfort.

CLINICAL CHARACTERISTICS

The patient presents himself to the physician with one or more physical symptoms as his chief complaint. He may seem appropriately concerned about his physical complaint or he may seem relatively unconcerned, *la belle indifférence*. In any event, the patient naturally feels that he has some sort of physical illness which is producing the symptoms and he seeks a medical diagnosis and treatment.

In some cases, the aggregate of conversion symptoms forms a syndrome that is remarkably close to a known organic syndrome. In such cases, it can usually be ascertained that the patient has had ample opportunity to acquire detailed knowledge of the particular organic syndrome which is mimicked by the conversion disorder. Thus, a patient who had long experience as a neurologist's secretary was followed in a neurologic outpatient clinic with the presumptive diagnosis of multiple sclerosis. When, after several years of observation, it was noted that at no time had any objective signs of neurologic disease been elicited, the more probable diagnosis was felt to be conversion hysteria. The latter diagnosis was supported, but not conclusively proved, by noting that a particular symptomatic flare-up appeared to be precipitated by severe psychic stress and was alleviated concurrently with successful management of the associated emotional problem.

Accurate knowledge of organic illness is of course not limited to medical secretaries, nurses, technicians, medical students, and physicians. The patient who unconsciously closely simulates an organic illness may have acquired knowledge of it by past experience of illnesses in himself or in friends and relatives. Thus, a patient of limited education and no history of medical or paramedical work experience presented with a clinical syndrome that mimicked tetanus with remarkable fidelity. It was learned that in the recent past she had cared for a close relative who was stricken with tetanus. It must also be remembered that suggestible patients may be inadvertently cued to develop symptoms by the syndrome-minded physician who asks leading questions during the history taking.

Not infrequently it is immediately obvious that the conversion symptom or syndrome could not have been produced by any anatomic or physiologic abnormality. In such instances, the patient's concept of physical illness and hence his unconscious simulation of it are apt to be relatively primitive or inaccurate.

In addition to knowledge and/or personal experience concerning specific physical illnesses, other factors which influence symptom choice include the need to choose symptoms that symbolically express one or more aspects of the underlying emotional conflict. Sometimes this symbolic function of the conversion symptom reveals an identification of the patient with a loved one who had some or all of the symptoms presented by the patient. This is illustrated by the following case.

A middle-aged, married woman was admitted to the medical service because of moderately severe, almost constant abdominal pain of two years' duration. Because of the pain and generalized weakness, the patient had not been able to keep up with her housework and other duties. In the year prior to admission, the patient spent more and more time in bed. During this period she came to feel depressed and she "explained" her feelings of depression by stating that her illness had prevented her from keeping her house the way it should be and from doing all the other things she normally would do for her family.

Thorough diagnostic evaluation revealed no evidence of organic illness. There was also no evidence of a functional gastrointestinal disorder which might have produced abdominal pain. As part of the diagnostic work-up, psychiatric consultation was obtained.

During the interview with the psychiatrist, the patient commented that her symptoms began shortly after the death of her father. She did not know the name of her father's terminal illness but when she was asked to describe his illness experience and symptoms, especially those of the last weeks of his life, she used descriptive phrases and gestures which were virtually identical with those she had used in describing her own symptoms.

It was also learned that the patient had been very close to her father. He had been an important, perhaps central, figure in the family until his fatal illness. He had been a decisive person who was always available to the patient and others when family problems came up and he tended to give his opinions in clear, definite terms. With a hint of submerged guilt, the patient indicated that there was no one to take his place. Her husband, in contrast to her father, tended to be a soft-spoken person who never took sides in family disputes, and who tended to be neutral and to seek compromises.

The consultant discussed these findings with the referring physician and suggested the possibility that the conversion syndrome might well represent an unconscious need of the patient for her late father, a need which was accentuated by the fact that no one else in the family had taken over the role once filled by him. The physician then undertook partially to fulfill some of the patient's needs which had formerly been met by the patient's father. He had several talks with the patient in which he encouraged her to tell him about her home, her family, and any problems or issues which were of concern to her. In the course of these conversations, the physician was quite definite in expressing his opinions about various personal issues and did so in a manner not unlike that of the patient's father as described by the patient. Within several days the patient's abdominal pain had remitted, and the patient no longer felt tired and depressed. Following discharge, the patient returned to her out-of-state home but continued occasional contact with the physician for several months during which time she remained symptom free.

ASSOCIATED EMOTIONAL DISORDERS

In the preceding example, the conversion syndrome appeared to be related to associated depression which was defended against or partially "contained" by the physical symptoms. This formulation is suggested by the fact that the patient's illness began shortly after the death of her father, was associated with feelings of depression and chronic fatigue, and was apparently alleviated when the physician served as a partial, symbolic substitute for the lost person. In psychoanalytic terms, this therapeutic result could be called a "transference cure."

Ziegler et al, in their study of 134 patients with conversion disorders, observed that in 40 patients depressive features were present.[7] The mean age of these 40 patients was 46.9 years as compared with a mean age of 36.4 years for the remaining patients of their series. They also noted that those conversion syndromes characterized by pain tended to occur in this subgroup and it was their impression that the conversion pain tended to mask signs of depressive illness. Conversely, the same investigators found that of 100 patients who were suffering from overt depressive illness, 28 patients also had conversion symptoms which almost invariably included pain. The association of conversion pain and depression has important treatment and management implications. These authors noted, for example, that even when the conversion symptoms substantially mask signs of depressive illness the suicidal risk is often considerable.

Conversion symptoms also may be associated with a variety of other emotional disturbances such as anxiety or, as illustrated by the following case, incipient schizophrenic disorganization.

A young, unmarried soldier was referred to the neurology clinic because of the sudden onset of deafness. The examining physician demonstrated the physiologic intactness of the auditory apparatus to his own satisfaction and then demonstrated to the patient that his deaf ear was actually functioning. (Such a demonstration does not, by any means, prove malingering. For example, electroencephalographic evidence of visual activity in conversion blindness is to be expected, and merely underscores the fact that conversion-based loss of function is on a psychologic basis and that objective physiologic signs have thus far not been found.) Following this demonstration that there was "nothing wrong" with his hearing, the patient was ordered to return to duty. The next day, the patient was found wandering in the desert several miles from his base. He was admitted to a nearby psychiatric facility where it was found that the patient was experiencing auditory hallucinations and showed other evidence of schizophrenic illness.

Patients with conversion hysteria or Briquet's syndrome have a history of chronic or recurrent, multiple somatic symptoms which began in adolescence or young adulthood. These patients are almost exclusively females and the somatic symptoms observed in them may include not only conversion symptoms but also a variety of other symptoms such as nausea, vomiting, dysmenorrhea, menstrual irregularity, frigidity, and dyspareunia. The patient typically has a long, complicated medical history, sometimes is under the care of several specialists at the same time, each of whom may have prescribed medications, and often has undergone a number of surgical procedures. Some, but not all, patients with conversion hysteria tend to be rather histrionic in their dealings with others, including physicians, and may be dependent, seductive, emotionally labile, and manipulative. It is not uncommon for these patients to have periods of being overtly anxious or depressed.

DIAGNOSIS

The diagnosis of conversion disorder is based upon (1) the probable exclusion of an organic basis for the symptoms and (2) supportive positive psychologic and historic evidence.

Since it is never possible to exclude organic disorder with absolute certainty, the clinician is compelled to pursue diagnostic evaluation until he can reach a judgment that organic disease is sufficiently improbable and that further testing is not indicated. In patients with conversion symptoms the physician notes whether there are objective signs of illness (signs which are very likely not reproducible by unconscious or conscious volition) such as absent or asymmetric deep tendon reflexes, abnormal reflexes, pupillary changes, fever, and so forth. The absence of objective signs of illness relevant to the particular symptoms or syndrome under investigation supports the diagnosis of conversion disorder. Closely related to this is the observation that the characteristics of the particular loss or disorder of function do not conform to known anatomic or physiologic principles. In the syndrome of astasia-abasia, for example, the patient is unable to stand or walk although motor strength of the legs and all modalities of sensation are normal. A more common example is that of cutaneous anesthesia whose distribution does not conform with that required by a peripheral or central lesion.

The diagnosis of conversion disorder receives support if (1) there is evidence that the illness began in association with psychic stress, (2) there is current evidence of coexisting emotional illness such as depression or anxiety, and (3) there is a previous history of conversionlike symptoms or medical history compatible with that described for conversion hysteria.

DIAGNOSTIC PITFALLS

It is to be stressed that the diagnosis of conversion disorder is in part based on exclusion of organic disease and should not be made entirely on evidence of psychologic vulnerability. This is illustrated by the following case.

A young married man was admitted to the medical service because of severe epigastric pain that penetrated to the back. Extensive evaluation including upper gastrointestinal series revealed no evidence of organic lesion to explain the patient's symptom. Further, it was learned that the patient's pain began several days after he had witnessed at close range the murder of a relative who died of a gunshot wound in the upper abdomen. In view of these circumstances and the negative diagnostic work-up, the patient was tentatively considered to have a conversion disorder and psychiatric consultation was requested. On the day before the scheduled psychiatric evaluation, the upper gastrointestinal series was repeated and this time a posterior duodenal ulcer was visualized. The quality and radiation of the patient's abdominal pain were entirely in keeping with this new finding.

Occasionally the physician quickly concludes that the patient is suffering from a conversion disorder and is thereby led to request psychiatric consultation prematurely or to discontinue further medical evaluation at a point which is far short of what the patient considers to be thorough. This is a particularly critical issue if the patient has been to other physicians and clinics and has now selected a particular physician or diagnostic center "as a last resort." Such a patient understandably wants no stone to be left unturned and will feel angry and rejected if the physician gives the appearance of having reached a diagnostic conclusion prematurely.

A middle-aged woman was admitted to the neurologic service of a large center because of back pain of several years duration. She had been to numerous physicians and clinics in a vain search for diagnosis and treatment and looked upon the present admission as almost her final chance to find out the cause of her pain. The attending neurologist, following physical and neurologic examinations, tentatively concluded that the patient was probably suffering from psychogenic pain and

171

decided to schedule psychiatric evaluation immediately even though other diagnostic procedures were also planned. When the psychiatrist arrived in the patient's room, the patient angrily told him that in her opinion the neurologist had taken one look at her and decided that she was just "an old crock," a middle-aged spinster with a backache. The patient felt that her symptoms had not really been taken seriously and she made it clear that she had no interest in talking further with the psychiatrist.

It is possible that the outcome would have been different if the neurologist had pursued the "organic" evaluation further and had discussed the test results with the patient, soliciting her opinions and concerns about her condition, prior to suggesting that psychiatric consultation would be of assistance as part of the clinical assessment.

In proceeding with diagnostic evaluation, the clinician must also bear in mind that the presence of a conversion disorder, of course, does not confer immunity against a coexisting organic condition. Indeed, it is not unknown for the patient with conversion disorder to have a nucleus of organically caused physical symptoms around which a more elaborate syndrome has evolved through the development of conversion symptoms.

It is also true, of course, that sometimes the patient is subjected to unnecessary or hazardous diagnostic examinations or may even undergo medical or surgical procedures as a therapeutic trial or test. Such experiences tend to fixate in the patient's mind the notion that he has some kind of organic disease.

A not uncommon diagnostic pitfall is that of unwittingly suggesting symptoms to the patient by asking leading questions. Since some patients with conversion symptoms, especially those with conversion hysteria, are quite suggestible and are attracted to the "sick role," it is quite possible for the physician to help bring into being a particular syndrome that he was endeavoring to "rule out" through a series of inquiries.

It has been noted that in conversion disorders, the patient unconsciously simulates physical illness. In factitious disease, on the other hand, the patient knowingly and willfully induces symptoms in himself by such means as self-administration of insulin, inducing vomiting, or feigning fever by warming the thermometer. The malingerer consciously feigns illness often with some specific purpose in mind, such as to avoid court trial or to support litigation. More often than not, patients who feign illness or have factitious disease are emotionally disturbed and need psychiatric evaluation.

MANAGEMENT

From the foregoing considerations, it is clear that diagnostic evaluation and management, as is so often the case, are closely interwoven. It is important for the physician to establish rapport and maintain communication with the patient as the diagnostic evaluation proceeds. The physician implicitly conveys to the patient that he is taking the patient's complaints seriously, reveals to the patient that thus far the examinations have not revealed the existence of this or that organic condition to explain the symptoms, asks the patient to express any specific theories or fears he may have about his condition, and begins tactfully to encourage the patient to talk freely about any present or past issues that might be disturbing to his sense of well-being. In initiating the latter phase of the inquiry the physician matter-of-factly explains that emotional problems not uncommonly manifest themselves in very real physical discomfort. By proceeding in this fashion, the physician will usually find that the patient becomes able to accept psychiatric consultation as a logical part of the overall evaluation and will not feel dumped or rejected. This is not to say that the primary physician or the psychiatrist will not encounter some degree of resistance to the exploration of psychologic issues or feelings, since the conversion symptoms themselves represent defenses against anxiety, depression, or some other dysphoric affect.

There are several approaches to treatment which may be utilized by the psychiatrist or the primary physician or both.

The patient with acute conversion symptoms often responds to a combination of suggestion and verbalization of the underlying psychologic problems. Suggestions should be employed with a degree of subtlety, the therapist being careful to avoid putting the patient in a position of losing face if he relinquishes his symptoms. In the following example, suggestion of symptom remission was used concomitantly with encouraging the patient to reverse the conversion process, ie, to substitute verbal expression of her problems and feelings for somatic expression of them.

The patient, a young housewife and mother, developed total body anesthesia, paralysis of all extremities, and loss of her voice while recuperating from an acute, febrile upper respiratory illness. After careful evaluation, the diagnosis of conversion disorder was made. In the first interview, the patient communicated with the psychiatrist by whispering. The psychiatrist encouraged her to review the development of her symptoms. He then indicated that it was not uncommon for persons under severe stress to develop the kinds of symptoms which she now had. He further indicated in a matter-of-fact way that, fortunately, symptoms such as these usually began to improve shortly after coming into the hospital. He wondered (aloud) if the patient was already able to wiggle her toes. She was. He then indicated that she would probably notice the feeling coming back in her arms and legs as well as the ability to move them in the next day or so. The psychiatrist then wondered what kind of stress the patient might have recently experienced. The patient, in the course of several interviews, described a severely disturbed marital situation which had culminated in an acute crisis the day before she became paralyzed and lost her voice. During these interviews the patient became able, with gentle suggestion, to speak in a normal voice and regained body sensation and full use of her extremities. Psychotherapy was continued for some months on an outpatient basis. It became clear that the acute conversion episode represented symbolically the patient's feeling that she had no voice in her marriage, that she felt unable to stand up for herself, was helpless, and wanted someone to take care of her.

In some instances an acute conversion episode evolves into chronic disability because of secondary gains or rewards for being ill that come to the patient from her environment. In this instance chronicity of the disorder develops even if the original psychologic stress or problem has been resolved. In this circumstance, a form of behavior modification in which symptom remission or return of function is systematically reinforced may be quite effective.

In those instances in which the conversion disorder is associated with some other psychiatric illness such as depression or schizophrenia, treatment is usually focused primarily on the associated disorder. For example, the patient whose conversion symptom such as pain appears to be associated with depression may respond to a combination of antidepressant medication and psychotherapy.

A common management error in patients with conversion disorders results from failure to diagnose the condition, with the result that these patients frequently have a history of excessive treatment with drugs and surgical procedures. As already noted, patients with conversion hysteria or Briquet's syndrome often have a history of polysurgery, excessive medication, and may sometimes receive more or less concurrent treatment from physicians in several specialties. The family physician plays a central role in coordinating management of these patients and thus in preventing duplicated or otherwise unnecessary diagnostic procedures, medications, and surgery.

Another type of management problem occurs when the physician reacts with anger or resentment toward the patient with conversion disorders. This kind of reaction is especially apt to occur if the physician regards the patient as a phony or malingerer. Whatever the source of the resentment, it too often may be expressed in overtly rejecting behavior or may lead the physician to overcompensate and thus be subject to manipulation by the patient. In the long-term management of patients with conversion hysteria it is therefore useful for the physician to have available a colleague with whom to discuss his feelings and experiences.

HYPOCHONDRIASIS

CLINICAL CHARACTERISTICS

Hypochondriacal neurosis is characterized by (1) a persistent preoccupation with bodily sensations and multiple symptoms which are often vague and involve several systems of the body, and (2) a conviction that the body

174

sensations and symptoms with which the patient is preoccupied indicate the presence of organic disease. This combination of features leads the patient to repetitive visits to physicians and clinics and to varying degrees of disappointment and resentment or bitterness over the failure of physicians to detect the elusive physical disorder and alleviate the patient's suffering. Some hypochondriacal patients strike the observer as being in the role of long-suffering martyrs who perceive themselves as persons who have been self-sacrificing for the sake of others. Patients with this condition are sometimes controlling in their relations with others, and may try to influence the physician to try this or that diagnostic test or therapeutic procedure. On the other hand, some hypochondriacal patients are rather passive in their dealing with others, including the physician. Regardless of the features of controllingness versus passivity, it is characteristic of hypochondriacal patients not to respond to reassurance about their physical health, even when this reassurance is based upon exhaustive medical evaluation.

Although a valid distinction can be drawn between hypochondriasis, conversion disorders, and psychophysiologic symptoms, one does encounter patients who exhibit features of all three of these conditions over a period of time.

DIAGNOSIS

The diagnosis is usually readily made on the basis of the characteristic, persistent preoccupation with bodily sensations, multiple symptoms, and failure to respond to the reassurance afforded by lack of evidence of organic disease when appropriate medical evaluation has been accomplished. The following psychiatric conditions, however, should be ruled out because of their obvious prognostic and management implications:

1. Temporary or transient hypochondriacal behavior. It is not uncommon for persons to develop transient, exaggerated concerns about physical health and a heightened sensitivity to bodily sensations and insignificant symptoms when under severe emotional stress. This transient state is not rare in patients who are convalescing from a serious physical illness and who may be hyperalert to minor symptoms which may be fearfully interpreted as indicative of return or persistence of the original illness.

2. Depression. It is not uncommon for depressed patients to develop a variety of physical complaints including various aches and pains, fatigue, anorexia, weight loss, and constipation. In psychotic depression there may be somatic delusions which can be interpreted as having self-debasing content. The diagnosis is made by discerning the presence of features associated with the depressive syndrome such as history of loss preceding onset of present illness, affect of sadness,

    self-deprecatory attitudes, pessimistic view of the future, and so forth (see Chap. 14).

3. Schizophrenia. Occasionally schizophrenic illness may be manifested early in its course or later by hypochondriacal behavior. In this condition, the hypochondriacal complaints may be a manifestation of somatic delusions. Schizophrenic illness is particularly to be suspected when the apparent hypochondriacal syndrome begins in adolescence or young adulthood or when there is a history of a prior psychotic episode.

MANAGEMENT

While it is true that at this time our knowledge of how to manage the hypochondriacal patient effectively is quite limited, it would appear that these patients can be helped and that in most cases the primary physician is in a better position to manage the patient than is the psychiatrist. The nature of hypochondriacal illness is such that the patient is apt to decline referral to the psychiatrist for treatment.

In his excellent discussion of hypochondriasis, Altman cautioned the physician against the tendency, on the one hand, to ignore the patient's emotional illness and to engage in unnecessarily extensive work-ups and procedures and, on the other hand, to attempt to persuade the patient that there is nothing wrong with him physically and that his trouble is entirely emotional.[1] It is important for the treating physician to keep in mind that the hypochondriacal patient apparently has a need to be preoccupied with physical symptoms and concerns about physical illness, and to accept his relationship with the patient on these hypochondriacal terms. The physician recognizes that the patient's symptoms are serving defensive purposes and are yielding the patient some gratification of needs for attention and dependency in his relationship with the doctor while at the same time protecting his self-esteem. If the physician does not expect early symptomatic remission both he and the patient will be less subject to the strain imposed by disappointment and frustration. As Altman has said, the goal of treatment is to allow the patient to maintain his hypochondriacal defenses while minimizing his suffering and his use of medical services.[1]

The physician's therapeutic approach is essentially a supportive one in that the patient is seen for brief sessions, perhaps 20 minutes or so, which are scheduled in advance and are therefore not contingent upon symptomatic exacerbation. During these sessions, the physician listens to the patient's description of how he feels, which will usually include a symptom recital, and concludes the session by a brief physical examination. The physician does not insist to the patient that he has no organic disease, but he may indicate that he finds no evidence that points to a specific physical disorder. This may be especially important to the patient who has some specific concern such as the possibility of having cancer. The physician couples his statement about the lack of organic findings with an indication that he realizes the patient is having uncomfortable symptoms and is worried about his health.

In the course of time, the patient may begin to mention various life experiences or current problems which are of concern to him. The physician responds to these excursions into psychologic issues by a show of interest but is prepared for the patient to return to somatic defenses as the need arises. The self-sacrificing type of patient may respond to the physician's appreciation of some example of self-sacrificing behavior which he chooses to describe. Similarly, the patient who needs to be in control of situations may respond to the physician's seeking his opinion about such matters as the frequency of visits or other aspects of management.

Considerable caution should be exercised in the prescription of minor tranquilizers for hypochondriasis because of the chronicity of the disorder, the dependency of the patient, and the doubtful efficacy of these drugs in this condition.

REFERENCES

1. Altman N: Hypochondriasis. In Strain JJ, Grossman S (eds): Psychological Care of the Medically Ill. New York, Appleton, 1975
2. Breuer J, Freud S: Studies on Hysteria. Standard Edition of the Complete Psychological Works of Sigmund Freud, Vol. 2. London, Hogarth, 1955
3. Chodoff P, Lyons H: Hysteria, the hysterical personality, and "hysterical" conversion. Am J Psychiatry 114:734, 1958
4. Purtell JJ, Robins E, Cohen ME: Observations on clinical aspects of hysteria. JAMA 146:902, 1951
5. Woodruff RA Jr, Clayton PJ, Guze SB: Hysteria. Studies of diagnosis, outcome, and prevalence. JAMA 215:425, 1971
6. Ziegler F, Imboden JB: Contemporary conversion reactions. II. A conceptual model. Arch Gen Psychiatry 6:279, 1962
7. Ziegler F, Imboden JB, Meyer E: Contemporary conversion reactions. A clinical study. Am J Psychiatry 116:901, 1960

Chapter

14

Mood Disorders

Management of the Depressed Patient
  Hospitalization
  Outpatient Treatment
    CHEMOTHERAPY
    PSYCHOTHERAPY
Mania
  Alteration of Mood
  Hypertalkativeness
  Hyperactivity
  Diagnosis and Management

Of the two major disorders of mood, depression and mania, depression is by far the more common.

Depression is one of the most common, serious disorders to affect mankind; the lifetime likelihood for anyone in the population to have a depressive illness is in the neighborhood of 5 to 10 percent. The ratio of depressed females to males is about 2 to 1. Although depression can occur in the very young it is primarily a disorder of adulthood, probably reaching its peak incidence in the fifth to seventh decades of life. The toll exacted by depressive illnesses in terms of human suffering, functional impairment, and economic loss is unquestionably enormous though difficult to measure. The lifetime risk of completed suicide among depressed patients has been estimated to be about 15 percent.[3]

THE DEPRESSIVE SYNDROME

Depression may occur in the apparent absence of a precipitating event but not infrequently its onset follows a psychologically stressful event within a few days or weeks. The type of antecedent stress is frequently of a sort that involves a loss of some kind, such as that posed by separation or divorce, death or serious illness of a loved one, moving to a new place of residence or to a new job, failure to perform satisfactorily at work or school with consequent loss of status or loss of certain hopes for the future, decline in ability to function as a result of illness or aging, and so forth. It is of practical and theoretical importance that some depressive illnesses continue long past the time when one would expect the patient to be getting over the effects of the disappointment or loss. In these cases it is as though the depression, though apparently precipitated by the "loss," continues autonomously just as aspiration pneumonia, which begins when the patient is comatose, continues after the patient is fully awake.

The clinical manifestations of depression may be grouped as follows: (1) subjective change in mood, (2) characteristic attitudes toward the self, (3) characteristic attitudes toward the future, (4) psychomotor symptoms, and (5) physiologic symptoms and somatic complaints.

SUBJECTIVE CHANGE IN MOOD

Typically, the patient complains of feeling "low," "down," "despondent," "blue," "sad," "unhappy," or simply "depressed." It is of interest that some patients will not spontaneously complain of the change in mood but will readily and often tearfully acknowledge it when directly asked.

Others may tend to dismiss the depressed mood as unimportant by ascribing it to some other symptom such as pain or fatigue. In such a case, the patient may state, in effect, that anyone would feel unhappy or depressed if he constantly had a particular discomfort such as an ache or pain or fatigue. Such a patient, who thus tends to minimize the subjective mood change of depression, may unknowingly mislead the physician diagnostically.

Still other patients seem to have little or no feeling of sadness even though they show other signs and symptoms of severe depression.

Frequently, the mood change and other symptoms of depression show diurnal variation, being worse in the morning than later in the day.

ATTITUDES TOWARD THE SELF

In mild depression, characteristically depressive attitudes toward the self may be sufficiently subtle as to escape discernment in a single interview. With increasing severity, however, the patient manifests unmistakable, highly characteristic attitudes toward himself which take the form of feeling that in one or more ways he has failed to live up to certain standards that he has set for himself. The patient may feel that his relatives and associates share his conviction that he is a failure or, alternatively, he may feel that others would share this perception of himself if they really knew him. The latter notion is often accompanied by the feeling that he has been a phony who has gone through life giving people a false impression of himself.

Typically, the patient conceives of his personal failure as stemming from (one or both) inadequacy and immorality. Thus, the patient may express conviction that he has mismanaged his business; that he is woefully lacking in those qualities necessary to being an adequate spouse, parent, friend, or professional; that he has no stamina; and that he lacks the strength of his convictions or that he has no convictions. Some investigators have observed that it is extremely common for the depressed patient to view himself as a "loser," and that this self-perception is often manifested in dreams as well as in the patient's statements.

Notions of being a failure morally are common among depressed patients. The associated feelings of guilt may be rather vaguely rationalized or they may be "explained" on the basis of some "sinful" or immoral behavior, which may strike the observer as being relatively trivial or as having occurred so far in the past that current reactions of guilt seem inappropriate. On the other hand the guilt feelings may be associated with global assertions by the patient that he has been greedy, selfish, inconsiderate of others, incapable of love, and so forth.

The perceptions of the self as inadequate, immoral, or both may be so obviously inappropriate and rigidly held as to clearly constitute delusional thinking. In extreme cases self-debasing attitudes may be presented in the form of gross distortions of body image or somatic delusions. Thus, the patient may have a delusion that his abdominal cavity is empty ("no guts"), his cerebral cortex is necrotic, feces is excreted from the pores in his skin, or he may state that he now sees himself as dirty or ugly when he looks in the mirror. In a peculiarly grandiose way, he may feel guiltily responsible for the misfortunes of others such as the illnesses of other patients on the ward.

ATTITUDES TOWARD THE FUTURE

In varying degrees, the depressed patient has a pessimistic and fearful attitude toward the future.

The patient's pessimism may involve his own illness which he may recognize as being a depression, it may involve some particular symptom such as pain or fatigue, or it may involve one of his fear-laden worries. It is not rare for the patient's pessimism to progress to the point of utter hopelessness. Thus, the patient may feel that he is beyond help, that he is condemned to feeling miserable for the rest of his life, or that one of his worst fears is going to be realized. Patients who feel severely depressed invariably think about death, usually wish for death, and if hope has been replaced by despair, may intend to commit suicide. The assessment of the patient's hopefulness versus despair and passive wishes for death versus active planning to suicide is critically important to management.

It is sometimes clear that the patient's attitude of despair is related to his self-concept as previously described. Thus, the patient who feels intensely guilty may feel that he deserves to suffer even more than he already has. Expectation of punishment may reinforce the patient's fear that some misfortune or catastrophe will happen to him or his loved ones, such as business failure, getting fired, sickness, and accidents.

PSYCHOMOTOR SYMPTOMS

Decline in interest, inability to experience pleasure, decrease in energy, and chronic fatigue are common features of depression. The patient may note that tasks which normally are easy and routine now seen difficult and burdensome.

Psychomotor retardation frequently occurs in severe depression and refers to a condition in which the patient feels mentally sluggish and is slow to respond to stimuli, both verbally and nonverbally. Speech may be sparse and in a low tone. The patient finds it difficult to concentrate, to take the initiative, and to make decisions. Productivity at home and at work markedly declines. Psychomotor retardation may progress to the point at which the patient becomes almost totally unresponsive and virtually mute, the so-called depressive stupor.

Agitation is sometimes observed in depressed patients. It is possible for the same patient to show predominantly agitation at one time and retardation at another. Agitation may take the form of relatively mild, transient periods of restlessness or relentless pacing back and forth, handwringing, and anxious, clinging behavior.

PHYSIOLOGIC ACCOMPANIMENTS AND SOMATIC COMPLAINTS

In addition to psychomotor activity, several other bodily functions are frequently affected in depression, especially sleeping, eating, sexual activity, and bowel function. Insomnia is very common in depression and is often characterized by awakening earlier than usual; difficulty in getting to sleep and sleeping fitfully throughout the night are not unusual. Hypersomnia is occasionally seen. Anorexia and consequent weight loss are frequent accompaniments of depression. Sexual difficulties may range from loss of interest in sex, which seems to be part of a generalized loss of interest in normal pleasurable activities, to erectile impotence. The latter symptom, which many patients do not mention unless asked, may cause the patient considerable worry. Constipation is commonly present in depression.

Various aches and pains may occur in depression and may affect virtually any part of the body, eg, feelings of heavy pressure over the chest, abdominal pain, headaches, backaches.

When physical symptoms are prominent, the patient and physician may understandably focus on serious organic possibilities before the diagnosis of depression is established. This is particularly apt to occur when the depressive mood is minimized by the patient or is dismissed as merely secondary to some other complaint. The patient with vague abdominal discomfort, chronic fatigue, anorexia, and recent severe weight loss poses a serious diagnostic challenge.

CLASSIFICATION OF DEPRESSIVE DISORDERS

The classification of depressive disorders has been a matter of debate for many years. A relatively simple system is that of classifying all primary depressions (those in which there is no other preexisting psychiatric disorder) into bipolar depression or unipolar depression. Bipolar depressions are those in which there is a history of one or more manic episodes. Unipolar depressions are those in which there is no history of manic episodes.

Unipolar depression is further classified according to whether there is a prior history of other episodes of depression. Thus, there is unipolar depression, single episode, or recurrent unipolar depression.

There is far less agreement on the classification of unipolar depression into further subtypes. Some investigators, for example, have contended that the distinction between reactive and endogenous depressions is not a valid one. However, we share the opinion of those who feel that at this stage of our knowledge such a distinction is useful.

By reactive depression, we refer to those depressed states which appear to be a response to some situational stress or loss. An example is the patient who has a grief reaction to a recent loss. Generally, reactive depressions tend to improve (though not necessarily to complete remission) with the passage of several weeks to two or three months. Further, patients with reactive depression are more apt to respond, though transiently at first, to favorable environmental circumstances and to psychotherapy, ie, their depressed mood is relatively less fixed and less subject to regular diurnal variation. The reactive depression is usually not accompanied by severe functional disability such as that which accompanies psychomotor retardation.

The endogenous depressions, on the other hand, appear to be relatively autonomous. That is, the patient's condition seems disproportionate to the precipitating event in both severity and duration. Autonomy is further marked by the relative lack of reactivity to daily events: environmental events or circumstances do not have much effect on how the patient feels and psychotherapy (alone) does not seem effective. However, diurnal variation in depressed mood and other symptoms is characteristically present. Psychomotor symptoms seem to be more prominent in endogenous than in reactive depressions, eg, loss of interest, anhedonia, psychomotor retardation, and agitation.

It has been suggested that depressions can be divided into neurotic or psychotic types. The validity of this distinction has been seriously questioned. At this time it may be more useful simply to estimate the degree of the depression and to use such adjectives as mild, moderate, or severe. Admittedly, it is difficult to give a precise definition of grades of severity.

It is worth noting that the old term, involutional melancholia, is still used. However, it has not been demonstrated that depressions occurring for the first time in the involutional period of life merit a separate category.

ETIOLOGY OF DEPRESSION

In considering the etiology of depressive disorders, one must keep in mind the likelihood that further research may ultimately show that these disorders comprise a more heterogeneous group than is indicated by their classification discussed above. At this time, clinical, laboratory, and family studies point to three sets of causative factors: psychologic, biochemical, and hereditary.

PSYCHOLOGIC FACTORS

An extensive literature has developed in which various psychodynamic concepts of the pathogenesis of depression have been elaborated.[1,5] Prominent among these concepts, the following have been implicated in attempts to understand depression: (1) reaction to loss, (2) loss of self-esteem, (3) inwardly turned anger, (4) insatiable demands for love, and (5) some combination of the foregoing.

Reaction to Loss　　It has been repeatedly observed that depressed patients frequently have experienced a loss prior to the onset of illness. Further, there is evidence, though admittedly not conclusive, that depressed patients more frequently have a history of significant loss early in life than do persons who are not prone to depression. This observation has given rise to the postulate that the earlier loss was never adequately resolved psychologically and, as a result, losses in later life serve to mobilize grief of childhood origin. The patient thus may be said to have been "sensitized" to experiences of loss by virtue of that which he experienced in childhood.

Inwardly Turned Anger　　The empiric observation that depressed patients are often quite self-derogatory and sometimes commit suicide led to the notion that depression could be explained as a psychologic phenomenon in which the patient is angry and directs his anger against himself. This postulate can be combined with that in which object-loss is implicated by considering that if loss has occurred or is threatened the person is apt to react toward the love-object with anger. If angry feelings toward the love-object are unacceptable to the patient he may then direct his criticism and rage toward himself. It can be seen that if the loss has not occurred but is only threatened, such self-direction of anger might serve to prevent disruption of the relationship between the patient and the love-object.

Loss of Self-Esteem   We have noted that many depressed patients look upon themselves as failures. Paradoxically, many observers have noted the frequency with which these patients have in fact been notably successful in their professional or business careers and in other aspects of their lives. From these and other observations it has been postulated that some depression-prone persons seem to feel that their lovability or acceptability is conditioned upon their constantly proving themselves to be worthy of love and acceptance by being successful. This puts the patient in the position of constantly looking to others for approval as though his independent approval of himself is lacking or does not matter. In this situation, the patient tends to interpret signs of disapproval or loss of love as meaning that he is an utter failure or, conversely, that if his performance is not sufficiently good he feels unlovable. In addition, some depression-prone patients seem to set such excessively high standards for themselves that they seem destined repeatedly to fail, at least in their own eyes.

Insatiable Demands for Love   It was noted in Chapter 2 that the mother's expression of love for her infant or child is intimately connected with the manifold ways in which she takes care of him. Deprivation of mother-love or prolonged, excessive indulgence or a combination of these can result in the child, and later the adult, developing an insatiable demand for mothering, ie, being cared for, attention, signs of approval, and so forth. When these "oral" demands are excessive, frustration and consequent rage are inevitable. The excessively demanding person tends unconsciously to alienate others because of his demandingness, while at the same time being particularly vulnerable to the effects of alienation.

BIOCHEMICAL FACTORS

The advent of psychopharmacology has stimulated intensive and promising research into the possibility that metabolic or biochemical factors play a critical role in the pathogenesis of the affective disorders. Biochemical observations, theories, and literature related to depression are complex and extensive. We will, however, confine ourselves to a brief consideration of the possible role of alterations in the availability of CNS neurotransmitters in depression, particularly the biogenic amines, serotonin and norepinephrine.[4]

Two observations originally suggested that a decrease in biogenic amines might be implicated in depression: (1) some patients receiving reserpine become depressed; reserpine administration is associated with depletion of CNS serotonin and the catecholamines; and (2) administration of iproniazid to tuberculosis patients who happened to be depressed resulted in substantial improvement in the depression; iproniazid is a monoamine oxidase (MAO) inhibitor which slows the rate of metabolic destruction of the biogenic amines.

Since these observations, further evidence has been obtained which supports, but does not prove, the biogenic amine depletion theory of depression.

1. In some depressed patients there is lowered urinary excretion of 3-methoxy-4-hydroxyphenylethylene glycol (MHPG); urinary excretion of MHPG is thought to be correlated with the concentration of norepinephrine in the brain.
2. In addition to MAO inhibitors, a group of drugs which have come to be known as the "tricyclic antidepressants" have been demonstrated to be effective in alleviating depression; these drugs inhibit the reuptake of serotonin or norepinephrine or both in the synaptic cleft, thus elevating the amounts of these neurotransmitters at the receptor site.
3. Similarly, dextroamphetamine, which inhibits reuptake of norepinephrine, is effective in temporarily alleviating depressive mood in patients whose urinary excretion of MHPG is below normal.

It is to be noted that correlation of CNS serotonin and/or norepinephrine levels with depression does not necessarily indicate a direct causal relationship between the two. It is possible, for example, that the ratio between cholinergic and noradrenergic levels of activity may be implicated in depression. It is possible that endocrine activity, electrolyte changes, neurophysiologic mechanisms involving the limbic system, or some factor still completely unknown to us may be implicated in depression.

HEREDITARY FACTORS

Family studies have shown that the occurrence of affective illness is significantly higher among the relatives of patients with bipolar and unipolar depressive illness than it is among the relatives of controls in whom there is no history of affective illness.[6] In the case of bipolar illness, the evidence to date is compatible with X-linked dominant transmission. Twin studies have indicated that the concordance rate in affective illness of monozygotic twins is substantially higher than that of dizygotic twins.

DIAGNOSIS OF DEPRESSION

Ordinarily the diagnosis of depression offers no particular difficulties. But nonetheless there are notable pitfalls which are particularly important to the primary physician since he is usually the first professional person to be consulted by the patient. Diagnostic errors can be made in both directions, depression being mistaken for some other entity and, less commonly, an organic medical disorder being mistaken for depression.

MASKED DEPRESSION

Masked depression refers to those instances in which the depressed patient minimizes the usual subjective mood changes of depression and focuses his complaints mainly on one or more somatic symptoms. For example, the patient may complain of abdominal discomfort, loss of appetite, and weight loss. Such a patient may blame his insomnia, tiredness, and general lack of energy on these complaints and attribute any recent tendency to feel downhearted (depressed) to his concern about the somatic complaints. It is to be emphasized that such patients may be genuinely unaware that their primary difficulty is depression and that they have "put the cart before the horse." In these sometimes very difficult cases, the diagnosis of depression is supported if careful reconstruction of the recent history reveals (1) that the present illness was preceded by a stressful life event of the "loss" type, and (2) that mood change, insomnia, and general decline in level of interest and activity were initial or early features and therefore probably not secondary phenomena. The diagnosis is also supported by a previous history of depression and a positive family history of affective illness. Careful physical evaluation is of course essential to rule out organic medical disorder.

INTRA-ABDOMINAL NEOPLASM

Rarely, carcinoma of the pancreas, stomach, or colon can present with a full-fledged depressive syndrome. The reason for this unusual and fascinating phenomenon is completely unknown. In depressions occurring in middle-aged or older patients, especially if there is no history of prior depressive episodes, it is wise to make a careful inquiry into symptoms apt to be associated with intra-abdominal neoplasms and, when indicated, to carry out appropriate laboratory and radiologic studies.

OTHER MEDICAL DISORDERS ASSOCIATED WITH DEPRESSIONLIKE SYMPTOMS

A variety of medical disorders may give rise to symptoms which may resemble those of depression such as apathy, chronic fatigue, diminution of interest, physical and mental sluggishness, and restlessness. Mention was made in Chapter 5 of the pitfalls in diagnosing depression in patients undergoing hemodialysis who may be intermittently uremic. Other disorders which may be associated with depressionlike symptoms include hypothyroidism, hyperparathyroidism, hypoparathyroidism, hyperaldosteronism, Cushing's syndrome, systemic lupus erythematosis, and Addison's disease. In addition, it is to be noted that almost any serious medical disorder can itself constitute a psychologic stress, eg, threatening the patient with functional and/or cosmetic loss, to which the patient reacts by becoming genuinely depressed (see Chap. 3).

PSEUDODEMENTIA IN THE ELDERLY PATIENT

Cognitive functions are considerably more vulnerable to emotional stress in the aged than in middle-aged or younger individuals. The depressed elderly patient may thus have severe difficulty in concentration, may be relatively inattentive to his surroundings and to the events of his daily life, and may become disoriented as to time and place, particularly if he is in unfamiliar surroundings. His ability to carry out customary, everyday functions concerning personal and interpersonal needs may have declined dramatically, suggesting the "personality change" often observed with progressive organic brain disease. Usually, recognition of the depressive nature of "pseudodementia" is not difficult, the patient (1) exhibiting the usual symptoms of depression already described, and (2) having a history of having developed evidence of depression early in the present illness, prior to the onset of functional incapacity and disorientation. The reconstruction of the history is greatly facilitated by interviewing a relative or other person who has been closely associated with the patient. The diagnosis will be confirmed by restoration of function when treatment succeeds in alleviating the depression.

DRUGS IMPLICATED IN PRECIPITATING DEPRESSION

As was noted above, the administration of reserpine is sometimes associated with the development of depression, even when administered in the relatively small doses used in the treatment of hypertension. Other drugs which may be associated with depression include diazepam (Valium), propranolol, methyldopa, and clonidine. The corticosteroids, though often associated with the production of euphoria, may occasionally be implicated in the precipitation of depression. It is not uncommon for drug-induced depression to persist long after the drug has been discontinued, and in such instances the patient may well require appropriate chemotherapy and psychotherapy for the depression.

188

DIFFERENTIATION FROM OTHER PSYCHIATRIC DISORDERS

Depressed patients, as described above, are commonly beset with worries and fears, and they may anxiously wring their hands and pace the floor. In other words, anxiety is a frequent feature of depressive illness. Conversely, patients with anxiety neurosis may become depressed. The differential diagnosis between anxiety neurosis and depression depends in part upon the history, the former diagnosis being favored by a history of anxiety symptoms which antedate the appearance of depression. Depressive illness is supported if (1) symptoms of depression began prior to those of anxiety; (2) depressive mood, self-derogation, psychomotor retardation, insomnia, and anorexia dominate the present clinical picture; (3) there is a prior history of one or more episodes suggesting depression with relatively symptom-free intervals; and (4) there is a positive family history of affective illness. Similar considerations apply to differentiating primary depression from depressive symptoms arising secondarily in the course of chronic conversion hysteria (Briquet's syndrome), obsessive-compulsive neurosis, and other neuroses. Patients with schizophrenic illness may also become depressed. As a rule the differentiation between schizophrenia and depression is not difficult. The depressive syndrome is not characterized by the thinking disorder typical of schizophrenia. When the depressed patient has delusions and, more rarely, hallucinations, the content of them reflect his depressive notions of inadequacy, guilt, and dread or expectation of punishment. Schizophrenic disorders tend to be chronic though with periods of exacerbation and incomplete remission, as contrasted with the relatively discrete episodes of depressive illness. Schizophrenia usually has its onset in adolescence or young adulthood, whereas depression becomes more frequent with increasing age.

MANAGEMENT OF THE DEPRESSED PATIENT

The first decisions to be made by the primary physician, once he has diagnosed or strongly suspects depressive disorder, concern (1) hospitalization versus outpatient care and (2) psychiatric referral versus management by the primary physician. Psychiatric consultation can be utilized in making and implementing either or both of these decisions.

HOSPITALIZATION

Hospitalization is indicated when (1) there is evidence of serious, imminent suicidal risk; (2) the depression is severe as evidenced by such symptoms as profound psychomotor retardation, agitation, guilt, hopelessness, delusions, and anorexia with substantial weight loss; or (3) the patient has not responded to outpatient treatment. When hospitalization is indicated it is advisable to refer the patient to a psychiatrist for continued management.

OUTPATIENT TREATMENT

In the event that the decision is made to manage the patient on an outpatient basis, the physician may elect to manage the patient himself with or without psychiatric consultation, or he may refer the patient to a psychiatrist for continued management.

There are no rigid criteria on which to base this decision. In part this decision will be determined by whether the physician feels comfortable and confident in treating depression, by whether his professional schedule permits him to take the time necessary for adequate management of the depressed patient, and by the availability of a competent psychiatrist in or near the patient's community.

The decision is also influenced by clinical features of the individual patient. For example, it is prudent to refer the depressed patient who has a past history of mania to a psychiatrist since there is a possibility that the current depression may be followed by a manic episode, particularly with the administration of antidepressant drugs. Further, even when the depression appears to be of the unipolar type, the primary physician may prefer psychiatric referral if he is uncertain about the degree of severity, the danger of suicide, or the possible presence of complicating factors. For instance, if the physician suspects that a schizophrenic disorder is present or incipient it is advisable to refer the patient to a psychiatrist.

Management of the patient with a depressive illness always includes a psychotherapeutic component and frequently includes the use of an antidepressant drug. The following discussion will be based upon the assumptions that the primary physician is managing the patient and that the depression is of a unipolar type, uncomplicated by any other psychiatric disorder.

Chemotherapy   It is not always easy to decide when to prescribe an antidepressant drug. While these drugs are of demonstrated value, one's enthusiasm for them has to be tempered by the fact that double-blind studies have repeatedly shown that a substantial number of depressed patients improve in a matter of weeks with supportive psychotherapy alone. Further, the use of antidepressant drugs, like the use of all drugs, is not without the risk of adverse side effects or complications.

If the depression is of mild to moderate severity and particularly if it is of rather recent onset, ie, four weeks or less, it is probably wise to give the patient a trial of supportive psychotherapy without the use of drugs. The latter can later be added to the regimen if necessary. This approach is particularly advisable if the patient has experienced a significant loss or severe disappointment a few days to two or three weeks earlier, with the subsequent development of grief and other symptoms. Such a patient often responds to a supportive relationship in which he has an opportunity to discuss his feelings and problems.

On the other hand, if the depression is of four weeks duration or longer it may be wise to prescribe an antidepressant drug without delay; this is particularly advisable when the depression is of moderate or greater severity and when the endogenous features described above are present. The chemotherapy of depression is discussed in detail in Chapter 18.

Psychotherapy   A substantial number of depressed patients can be effectively treated with supportive psychotherapy without the use of drugs. As was previously noted, this particularly holds true for patients whose depression is relatively mild or of recent onset and is associated with a disturbing life event or situation such as separation, death, or serious illness in the family; vocational or business failure; and so forth. Persons who have recently suffered such misfortunes can, of course, be expected to grieve and, for some period of time, to have such symptoms as insomnia, decreased interest, and difficulty in putting their minds to everyday tasks. Sometimes, the "depressing" environmental factor does not consist of a recent discrete event but rather may be a continuing, unresolved issue that, one way or another, threatens the patient with a significant personal loss. In either case, the patient will benefit from regularly scheduled sessions, weekly or more often, in which he has the opportunity to express and discuss his feelings and ideas about himself and the important other people and issues in his current life situation.

The primary physician, as a person who is known and trusted by the patient, is in an excellent position to be the one to listen to the patient and to help him to accept the unchangeable aspects of reality and constructively approach those things which the patient can do something about. This supportive therapeutic approach, which requires a relationship characterized by interest and respect, need not and usually does not require interpretation of unconscious meanings and defenses. Further, the psychotherapeutic management of this type of depression in which there is predominantly a reactive component may require a fairly brief period of time such as two or three months. The individual sessions may also be relatively brief, eg, 30 minutes. The physician may or may not find it useful to suggest to the patient that a close family member be included in the therapy sessions from time to time or even on a regular basis. Some patients may welcome this while others will clearly wish and probably need to see the doctor alone for awhile.

As was indicated earlier, even when drug treatment is instituted the depressed patient still needs supportive psychotherapy.

In treating the severely depressed patient it is helpful to let the patient know that the physician appreciates that he feels pessimistic about his chances of ever feeling better. One can indicate to the patient that more often than not a person's outlook toward himself and toward the future is strongly influenced by the depressed state, and that it is therefore very common for a depressed person to feel inadequate or guilty or both and to feel pessimistic or frankly hopeless about his chances of getting well. One can then matter-of-factly inform the patient that depressions are treatable and that the prospects for recovery are excellent.

When the patient's illness is such that he feels tired, slowed down, or sluggish, it is advisable to spell out the treatment plan to him in a simple, clear fashion and to keep the therapy sessions relatively brief and frequent, such as 20 minutes twice a week.

The issue of suicidal risk is best managed by tactfully but forthrightly asking the patient if he has wished for death and if he has thought about or had intentions of ending his own life. Most depressed patients have transient wishes to die and have had at least the possibility of suicide occur to them. If however the patient expresses a suicidal intention, or expresses a fear that he may yield to an impulse to suicide, or if his behavior suggests suicidal intentions (such as recently procuring a revolver), psychiatric referral and hospitalization are indicated. In any event, when the physician makes such an inquiry he has an opportunity to let the patient know that he wishes to be kept informed about the patient's thoughts and feelings concerning death or suicide. Maintaining open communication about this matter is a much more effective approach to suicide prevention than silence.

MANIA

Reference has been made to bipolar depressions which by definition are characterized by a history of one or more episodes of mania. We will limit this discussion to a brief description of the salient clinical features of mania.[2]

Most of the characteristics of mania fall into three categories: alteration of mood, hypertalkativeness, and hyperactivity.

ALTERATION OF MOOD

Classically, the manic patient is euphoric. He may use any of a variety of adjectives to describe his euphoric mood: high, perfect, on top of the world, great, very happy, and the like. Occasionally the patient will attempt to explain his elevated mood by saying that he has had or is about to have some remarkable success such as an invention, a business venture, or a scientific discovery which will bring him fame and wealth. He may feel he has arrived and the world is his oyster. He can do anything or be anything he sets his mind to.

On the other hand, the manic patient typically tolerates frustration very poorly and may become dangerously enraged when thwarted. The euphoria may also give way to periods of irritability. It is not rare for the manic patient to be hostile or suspicious. Frank paranoid delusions are sometimes seen.

HYPERTALKATIVENESS

The manic patient talks excessively and rapidly. In milder cases, speech is more or less coherent and its content reflects the patient's euphoric mood, his grandiose concept of himself, and his accomplishments and plans. His speech may also reflect his anger at others who try to restrain him or his general irritability. In more severe mania, speech becomes very rapid, the patient frequently shifts from one line of associations to another, and he may engage in rhymes and puns or plays on words. This more severe speech disturbance is called "flight of ideas" and is virtually incomprehensible.

HYPERACTIVITY

The patient is full of energy and engages in all sorts of activities which, as in the case of his speech, reflect his euphoric mood and grandiosity. Often the patient's hyperactivity has a frenetic quality, the patient impulsively going from one thing to another, without adequate planning and often without follow through. Judgment is blatantly poor. The patient may go on a shopping spree, make travel plans, contact others regarding this or that grand venture, and so forth. Insomnia is common. It is not unusual for the manic patient to eat very poorly while at the same time expending a great deal of energy.

The term hypomania is often used and simply refers to mild mania. In very mild instances in which the patient has periods of feeling a bit elated and, while being more talkative and active than usual, does not seem obviously grandiose and does not behave impulsively or with poor judgment, the observer may be hard put to draw the distinction between normal mood swing and hypomania.

DIAGNOSIS AND MANAGEMENT

In most cases of mania of moderate to severe degree, the diagnosis is apparent and is made on the basis of the triad of features described above. The history of the patient's recent behavioral change must usually be obtained from a relative or friend. The patient himself as a rule has little or no insight into his illness and in fact usually considers that, if anything, he is superhealthy.

Occasionally the incoherence of speech and such features as suspiciousness or paranoid delusions may raise the question of a schizoaffective disorder. In any patient who is elated the physician must also consider the possibility of drug intoxication, and it is always wise to make a careful inquiry into the history of recent drug ingestion.

It is advisable for the primary physician to refer the patient who is hypomanic or manic or the currently depressed patient who has a history of manic episodes to a psychiatrist for evaluation and management.

Lithium carbonate is commonly employed by the psychiatrist in the management of a manic episode and for prevention of future episodes. The psychiatrist frequently requests medical consultation if there is any concern about the presence of medical contraindications to the administration of lithium carbonate. The administration of lithium carbonate and its side effects are discussed in Chapter 18.

REFERENCES

1. Beck AT: Depression. New York, Harper & Row, 1967
2. Cohen RA: Manic-depressive illness. In Freedman AM, Kaplan HI, Sadock BJ (eds): Comprehensive Textbook of Psychiatry, 2nd ed. Baltimore, Williams and Wilkins, 1975, Chap. 17.2
3. Guze SB, Robins E: Suicide and primary affective disorders. Br J Psychiatry 117:437, 1970
4. Maas JW: Biogenic amines and depression. Arch Gen Psychiatry 32:1357, 1975
5. Mendelson M: Psychoanalytic Concepts of Depression, 2nd ed. New York, Spectrum, 1974
6. Winokur G, Pitts FN: Affective disorder. VI. A family history study of prevalences, sex differences, and possible genetic factors. J Psychiatr Res 3:113, 1965

Schizophrenic Disorders

Management
Chemotherapy
Psychotherapy
Social Therapy

Schizophrenia refers to a group of conditions characterized by disturbances of thought, affect, and behavior that lead eventually to a wide
variety of signs and symptoms, such as social and emotional withdrawal,
mood disturbances, periods of excitement and immobility, misinterpreta-
tions of reality, delusions, and hallucinations. Although the constellation
of signs and symptoms comprising a schizophrenic syndrome is often
unmistakable, yet there is no single sign or symptom that is pathog-
nomonic of schizophrenic illness.

Schizophrenic illness usually begins during adolescence or young
adulthood. The incidence of new cases in the United States among people
age 15 and above is estimated at between 0.3 and 1.2 per 1000 per year.[3]
Because of the early age at onset, the seriousness of the disorder, and its
tendency to be chronic or recurrent, schizophrenic illness accounts for
one-third to one-half of the beds occupied in psychiatric hospitals. All
races and socioeconomic groups are affected, but the prevalence is higher
among the poor.

In recent years it has become increasingly important for the primary
physician to be familiar with these disorders. This is true for several
reasons. Since the advent of effective chemotherapy, more schizophrenic
patients are able to live outside the hospital. As a result, the physician is
now much more apt to be consulted in the clinic or in his office by the
schizophrenic patient who happens to have an incidental medical problem
or whose emotional disturbance manifests itself in somatic symptoms or
concerns. Further, potent chemotherapeutic agents, sometimes in very
high dose, are commonly used in the management of schizophrenic illness. The physician may be involved in the management of patients who
exhibit side effects or toxic reactions to these drugs. He must be knowledgeable of the condition for which these agents are used so that he may
have some idea of what to look for if chemotherapy must be discontinued.
Finally, and most importantly, it is usually the family physician to whom
the patient and/or his family first turn for help in the early stages of the
illness, and whose advice and counsel will continue to be sought during
the often prolonged course of psychiatric treatment.

ETIOLOGY

There is no single cause of schizophrenia. In the past, various theories of etiology have competed, but now, as with many other diseases, schizophrenia is considered to be the result of several interacting factors.

GENETIC FACTORS

Genetic studies have repeatedly indicated that the concordance for schizophrenia is significantly higher among pairs of monozygotic twins than among pairs of dizygotic (fraternal) twins. In addition, recent studies of schizophrenics who were adopted at birth into nonschizophrenic families have found higher incidence of schizophrenia among the biologic relatives (parents, siblings, or half-siblings) than among the general population.[7]

BIOCHEMICAL FACTORS

The genetic factor is probably mediated by a biochemical change or set of changes. Here, only hypothesis has so far been offered, with no clear proofs. For example, dopamine has been implicated in Snyder's hypothesis,[11] since phenothiazines and other antipsychotic medications block dopamine receptors (this probably accounts for the production of parkinsonism as a side effect). In addition, dextroamphetamine, which can exacerbate schizophrenic psychoses or induce a schizophrenialike illness when given in large doses, increases the activity of neurotransmitters at dopaminergic as well as noradrenergic synapses in the central nervous system.

EARLY ENVIRONMENTAL INFLUENCES

Family experiences during childhood no doubt sometimes play a part in the development of schizophrenia, but the clearcut descriptions of a decade ago of the schizophrenogenic mother or of specific pathologies in the families of schizophrenic patients have not held up. On the other hand, it does seem clear that such factors as marked parental inconsistency, ambiguity of communications with the child, and failure to provide adequate role models or an atmosphere of love and acceptance are all likely to impair personality development and thus intensify the stressfulness of life. This may be of great importance in the individual genetically predisposed to schizophrenic illness.

CURRENT STRESS

Stress resulting from current psychologic and social pressures frequently appears to play a role in schizophrenic decompensation. It has long been noted, for example, that the illness often makes its appearance at the transitional junctures of adolescence or young adulthood.

In sum, then, while etiology is far from fully understood, it does appear that the several factors of genetic predisposition, biochemical malfunctions, early environmental influences, and current stress all contribute to the development of schizophrenic illness.

CLINICAL CHARACTERISTICS

MODE OF ONSET

In some patients there is a preillness history of shyness, oversensitivity, emotional inhibition, and a tendency to daydream and to be a loner. Many patients, however, do not have such a history and many persons who do have such a history never become afflicted with a schizophrenic illness.[9]

The onset may be insidious, sometimes consisting initially in progressive withdrawal from friends and family, decline in academic interest and achievement, hypochondriacal preoccupations, multiple somatic complaints, and neurotic symptoms such as obsessions and compulsions. In this insidious mode of onset months may go by before the family realizes that something serious is going on, and this realization may not occur until some bizarre, disturbing behavior develops.

In other patients, the illness develops more rapidly and dramatically, the patient exhibiting such unmistakable evidences of profound disturbance as psychomotor excitement, panic, marked alteration of mood, delusions, and hallucinations.

The initial development and subsequent exacerbations of schizophrenic illness may or may not be associated with stressful events or situations. As already noted, often the illness tends to develop or worsen around transitional periods of youth: puberty, adolescence, graduation from high school or college, leaving home or school and facing the prospects of going out into the world.

DISTURBANCE OF AFFECT

The affective manifestations of schizophrenic illness are manifold and vary greatly from one patient to the next and in the same patient over a period

198

of time. Not infrequently the patient exhibits a reduction or "flattening" of affect: this feature may be associated with a progressive diminution or narrowing of interests and loss of ability to experience pleasure or deep satisfaction in any activity or interpersonal relationship. This anhedonic state often leads the patient to feel empty, isolated, and lost; he may despair of ever being better and may contemplate suicide. Affective flatness and withdrawal may make the patient seem exasperatingly indifferent to everything and everybody.

The patient may also display affect that seems silly or inappropriate to what he is talking about or to his situation. He may, especially early in the illness, have a burst of emotion accompanied by a sudden conviction that "everything is clear" about previously mysterious events.[1] The patient may have periods of melancholy, elation, irritability, anger, and fearfulness.

DISTURBANCE OF COGNITIVE FUNCTIONS

Evidence of cognitive disorder may be revealed in difficulties in communication, and in the development of delusions and hallucinations.

Communication   In normal communication, one attempts to convey a concept to the listener. In doing this, one must often relate background material or subordinate concepts in order to get the main idea across. Thus, normal communication requires the speaker, on the one hand, to be in touch with associations relevant to the idea he is communicating and, on the other hand, to screen out those which are irrelevant. In schizophrenic thought disorder there may be difficulty with either or both of these processes, ie, severe inhibition of associations or failure in screening out tangential and irrelevant associations. Both of these difficulties may result in speech that is poorly connected or fragmented, ie, in what is often referred to as "loosening" of associations.

When the associative processes are severely constricted the patient may find that his thoughts are frequently "blocked" so that he loses his train of thought. Constriction of associations may be revealed in a tendency to concrete thinking as manifested by very narrow, literal interpretations of simple proverbs. The patient may indicate that he feels he has no thoughts and may indicate that his thoughts have been taken from him by an outside agency.

On the other hand, failure to screen out irrelevant or tangential associations often occurs and may result in excessively circumstantial speech; in extreme cases, the patient never seems to get to the point—his speech is rambling, vague, and difficult or impossible to follow. He may be strikingly overinclusive when asked a straightforward question or when confronted with a simple task or problem.

Other disturbances of communication include the idiosyncratic use of words, creating new words (neologisms), repeating words or phrases in a stereotyped fashion, and negativism.[10]

Delusions   Everyone's judgment, beliefs, reasoning, and even perceptions are influenced to a degree by currently prevailing emotions, especially wishes and fears. In a state of intense fear, for example, one may interpret innocuous shadows and sounds as having some ominous significance. In patients with schizophrenic illness, cognitive functions may be abnormally vulnerable to such influences as wishes and fears.

Many schizophrenic patients tend to be preoccupied with the fear of being controlled or influenced by other persons or "outside forces." It is possible that in some cases this apparent fear represents an underlying wish. In any event it is not uncommon for the patient to express the notion that he is being kept under surveillance, is followed when he walks down the street, that thoughts are being inserted into or withdrawn from his mind, that his behavior is being directed by someone, that bodily sensations are being imposed upon him. He may have the delusion that he is being persecuted. The patient's delusions may be elaborate and well systematized (internally consistent) or they may be unelaborated or fragmented.

Preoccupation with the self, and absorption in his own fantasies and bodily processes are characteristically present. This narcissistic orientation in conjunction with defensiveness concerning feelings of loneliness, inadequacy, and guilt may lead to a variety of delusions. Notions of grandiosity are often seen, particularly in patients who feel they are the target of a conspiratorial plot. Ideas of reference occur in which the patient believes that he is the subject of news articles, television programs, and so forth. Somatic delusions, sometimes buried in what superficially looks like a hypochondriacal neurosis, are not rare.

Sometimes, the outer world seems distant, strange, and unreal (derealization) and sometimes he himself feels unreal (depersonalization). The patient may identify the cosmos with himself and, fearing the dissolution of his own mind, have the conviction that the end of the world is nigh.

Hallucinations   In schizophrenic illness, hallucinations involving any sensory modality may occur, but usually they are predominantly auditory. Auditory experiences of several types are found. Voices may be heard which are discussing the patient and which refer to him in the third person, or which describe or comment on the patient's activities as they take place. The patient may have the experience of hearing his own thoughts, as though aloud but within his head ("gedankenlautwerden").[10]

As one may infer from the above description of the profound disturbances in affect and cognition, schizophrenic patients may show a wide variety of behaviors which range from the mildly eccentric to the bizarre. Many schizophrenic patients are obviously ill at ease with other people and may seem awkward or gauche in social situations. An air of guardedness or suspiciousness is common in patients with paranoid tendencies. On the other hand, some schizophrenic patients may not reveal any particular behavioral clues of their illness in casual social situations, while nonetheless revealing unmistakable pathology when carefully interviewed or when observed over a period of time.

Particularly striking alterations of psychomotor behavior are catatonic stupor and catatonic excitement. In the former state the patient is immobile, sitting or standing in same position for hours, not speaking or eating; in catatonic stupor, the patient's hand or arm remains in the position in which it is passively placed (waxy flexibility). In catatonic excitement, the patient may lose control of aggressive impulses and may strike out suddenly at people and things in his immediate environment; the patient may be generally overactive, running around wildly and talking incoherently.

CLASSIFICATION

There are several ways of classifying the various subtypes of schizophrenia. We will consider only three.

THE CLASSIC SYNDROMES OF KRAEPELIN AND BLEULER

The syndromes of Kraepelin and Bleuler do not occur in as pure and stable a form as one would infer from the early descriptions of schizophrenia.[9,10] The comparative rarity of these syndromes "in pure form" is in part due to the influence of modern chemotherapy. The classic syndromes referred to are as follows.

Paranoid Schizophrenia   In paranoid schizophrenia, ideas of reference, delusions of being watched, followed, or persecuted, and delusions of grandiosity dominate the clinical picture. Onset of the illness tends to be somewhat later than in other forms of schizophrenia, often first becoming manifest in the 30s age group. These patients are often tense, guarded, and suspicious. Typically there is rather good preservation of intellectual function (outside of the delusions) and the patient may be able to function well in many areas of life.

Catatonic Schizophrenia   Catatonic schizophrenia applies to patients whose illness is primarily manifested by the disturbances in psychomotor behavior described above: catatonic stupor and/or excitement. In addition, catatonic patients typically have hallucinatory experiences and delusions as well as psychomotor symptoms.

Hebephrenic Schizophrenia   Hebephrenic schizophrenia typically begins in the teens (Hebe, the Greek goddess of youth). It is a severe disorder characterized by silly, inappropriate affect, hallucinations, poorly organized delusions, and severely regressive behavior.

Simple Schizophrenia   Simple schizophrenia is characterized primarily by *progressive* shallowness of emotion, and reduction in interests and in attachments to things, situations, and people. Patients with this condition show little interest in holding a job or pursuing goals. They may show little evidence of delusions and hallucinations.

PROCESS–NONPROCESS SCHIZOPHRENIA

It has been found useful to classify schizophrenic illness into two types: one characterized by features associated with a relatively good prognosis (nonprocess type), and the other by features associated with a relatively poor prognosis (process type.)[12]

The relatively good prognosis type is characterized by the following: good preillness level of adjustment, presence of stress at time of onset, acute onset, presence of excitement, tension, anxiety, and affective symptoms. Illnesses falling into the good prognosis group may be referred to as nonprocess schizophrenia, reactive schizophrenia, schizoaffective disorder, remitting schizophrenia, and schizophreniform illness.

The group with relatively poor prognosis is sometimes referred to as process schizophrenia or "true" schizophrenia and its characteristics are poor preillness adjustment; slow and insidious onset; absence of precipitating stress; relative lack of tension, anxiety, or affective symptoms; emotional blunting or flatness; and relatively high incidence of schizophrenic illness in the family.

It is important to note that when dealing with individual patients, the prognostic indicators noted above do not always prove to be accurate.[4] That is, it is imperative to proceed with active treatment and with a hopeful attitude regardless of which group the patient appears to belong to.

THE CLASSIFICATION OF KLEIN AND DAVIS

These investigators have offered a classification of schizophrenia based on presenting symptoms, childhood adjustment, and likely response to medications.[8] It has the virtues of simplicity and a close connection to the patients as we may encounter them in clinical practice. Klein and Davis have classified schizophrenic disorders into three groups as described below.

1. "Schizophrenia–childhood asociality" is a condition with marked thought disorder, much disorganized thinking (even delusions are vague), and fragmented verbal productions. In affect, these patients are frightened rather than angry or depressed. History of their childhood shows aloof, cold, asocial behavior, with no real friendships. This group of patients is the least likely to respond to treatment, and long-term prognosis is poor.
2. "Schizophrenia–fearful paranoid" presents with a suspicious and defensive patient, who has clear-cut delusions, ideas of reference, and paranoid ideas about other people. Delusions may include beliefs in changes in shape, size, or function of bodily parts. The patient may be depressed or suicidal, especially early in the course of illness. Angry outbursts may occur when the paranoid patient believes himself to be trapped. Childhood is typically not so disturbed, though there may be some pattern of being a loner. These patients are likely to respond to treatment, and the prognosis is fair to good.
3. "Schizophrenia–schizoaffective" refers to an illness with definite affective psychotic manifestations, resembling either mania or psychotic depression; in addition, the patient must show clear-cut schizophrenic thought disorder with bizarre and/or persecutory delusions. The illness is often of acute onset, and response to treatment is generally good with a favorable prognosis in the long run.

DIAGNOSIS

In its florid form, the diagnosis of schizophrenia usually presents no difficulty. In early stages of the illness, however, especially when the onset is slow and insidious, it may be extremely difficult to make a definite diagnosis until the patient has been observed over a period of time. In such instances, the initial manifestations may consist predominantly of neurosislike symptoms such as hypochondriacal preoccupations, obsessions, and compulsions, or a sort of social maladjustment with such features as decline in school performance, and a progressive tendency to withdraw from interpersonal contacts and to prefer solitary pursuits. Such symptoms occurring in an adolescent or young adult may arouse the suspicion of schizophrenic illness and lead the physician to be alert to the presence of the characteristic disturbances in cognition and affect, perhaps present in relatively subtle or mild form.

With regard to more fully developed schizophrenic disorder, it should be kept in mind that a variety of conditions can be associated with delusions, hallucinations, and other symptoms common in schizophrenia; among these are the organic brain syndromes and affective disorders.

Typically, in schizophrenic illness the sensorium is clear and if hallucinations are present it is common for the auditory type to be predominant. In delirium, in addition to clouded sensorium, visual hallucinations often predominate.

Hallucinations and delusions can occur in severe depressive and manic states; in that event their content usually reflects a depressive or expansive attitude toward the self and the future. Other manifestations of affective illness should be sought including a family history of affective illness.

Amphetamine intoxication can closely simulate schizophrenic illness; the diagnosis is made by a history of amphetamine ingestion and by relatively rapid (one to two weeks) symptomatic remission following separation from the drug, which is sustained for as long as the patient abstains from further amphetamine ingestion.

In the diagnostic evaluation of patients with schizophrenic illness, no matter how obvious the diagnosis appears, the physician conducts a careful neurologic and general medical examination just as he does in evaluating patients with other types of illness.

MANAGEMENT

The patient with schizophrenic illness should be referred to the psychiatrist for continued evaluation and treatment. This does not mean, however, that the primary physician will have no further role in the management of the patient. More often than not, worried parents will consult the primary physician from time to time, even after the psychiatric referral is made, in order to have his opinion about various aspects of the treatment and course of the patient's illness. The parents may feel guilty, as if they are to blame for their son's or daughter's illness, and seek the physician's counsel about their feelings. The parents and the patient may rely on the advice of the primary physician as to whether to accept some specific recommendation, such as hospitalization, that the psychiatrist may have made. For these and other reasons, it is appropriate for the physician to have some general understanding of the psychiatric management of schizophrenic illness, and for the primary physician and the psychiatrist to communicate with each other from time to time about the patient's treatment and progress.

Treatment for schizophrenic patients includes several modalities.[5] We have previously described patterns of symptoms and the most expected prognosis based on stereotyped descriptions. Now as we consider treatment of the individual patient, however, we are reminded that population statistics do not provide a valid ironclad predictor for outcome in any individual patient. Therefore, each schizophrenic patient should have a vigorous and thorough program of treatment, regardless of the characteristics of his particular illness.

The overall goals of treatment are reduction of the duration and degree of disability for each patient in each episode of illness, and limitation of the impact of the patient's illness on family and community. Subsidiary objectives in planning for these goals include reduction of psychotic symptoms, decreasing the disruption of personal life, and finding ways to prevent future relapses.

The means of treatment are a network or system of services. Just as the illness has developed within the context of a person's life, so treatment must be planned to fit into that context or skillfully to alter the context of the patient's life. Psychiatrists, psychiatric outpatient clinics, psychiatric hospital services, and social work and rehabilitation programs all collaborate in providing continuity of clinical services. A single person must coordinate these joint efforts; sometimes this person is the psychiatrist, sometimes the family physician.

Techniques of treatment can be divided into three categories: chemotherapy, psychotherapy, and social therapy.

CHEMOTHERAPY

Chemotherapy has become the mainstay of therapy for schizophrenia.[2,8] Antipsychotic drugs have been demonstrated as markedly more effective than placebos in promoting recovery from acute episodes of schizophrenic psychosis. Psychotic symptoms are disruptive to the patient and to those around him, and the judicious use of adequate doses of antipsychotic medications can do much to relieve the suffering.

A number of antipsychotic drugs are available, and their major actions are similar. Choice of a particular one depends on the secondary effects or side effects, and on the patient's responses. The less potent phenothiazines (Thorazine, Mellaril) are more sedating, and tend to have lower incidence of extrapyramidal side effects. Those which are more potent per milligram of dose are less sedating, and more likely to give some extrapyramidal side effects. The newer nonphenothiazine antipsychotics include butyrophenones (Haldol), thioxanthenes (Navane), dibenzodiazepines (Loxitane), and molindone (Moban). They are particularly useful in patients who do not improve on phenothiazines, or who have side effects or allergic reactions which dictate a change of medication.

One medication should be used at a time; polypharmacy is not generally helpful in chemotherapy of schizophrenia. The medication chosen should be given in adequate dosage for a long enough time to have a full effect. Since these medications have a half-life of over 24 hours, a single daily dose can be prescribed rather than the divided dosages necessary for shorter-acting drugs. Antipsychotic effects may occur within a few days, or may not become evident for several weeks. Dosages can be increased at three-day intervals, until the desired effect appears. See Chapter 18 for further discussion of antipsychotic drugs.

PSYCHOTHERAPY

Psychotherapy is another essential aspect of treatment of schizophrenic patients. A personal relationship between physician and patient, and the resultant issues of trust, responsibility, and influence, are of critical importance. While psychotherapy alone rarely is sufficient as a treatment for schizophrenia, the planned use of a human relationship can make a significant difference in the way a patient responds to the other components of the treatment plan.

Several purposes are served by the use of psychotherapy in schizophrenia.

1. A model for effective, clear communication with another person can be established and experienced.
2. When rapport and a degree of trust have been established, the therapist is in a position to assist the patient to improve his ability to test reality; this activity is best done in a fashion that encourages the patient to consider nonpsychotic interpretations of his experiences rather than one in which the therapist imposes his views on the patient.
3. The patient can receive necessary emotional support and encouragement.
4. Introspective patients can review their experiences in the postpsychotic phase of illness, to better understand and integrate their recent psychosis in the context of the rest of their lives.
5. Also in the postpsychotic phase, patients with depression can receive support and gain some comfort.
6. After a psychosis, patient and physician can examine the issues and conflicts that may have contributed to the development of a schizophrenic psychosis, with the aim of lessening the patient's vulnerability for another later psychosis. For example, a young woman who had had

two brief but severe schizophrenic psychotic episodes, both after romantic disappointments, was able to learn how she had picked men who would not carry out their end of the relationship.

In beginning psychotherapy the establishment of a trusting relationship is always paramount. This may be particularly difficult with a schizophrenic patient who is fearful, suspicious, and antagonistic. Nonetheless, the therapist can do several things that increase the opportunity for his patient to develop trust. Being open and straightforward is the most helpful attitude, since the patient can sense that he is being dealt with as an adult with rights and responsibilities. The therapist who is sincere, who explains things to his patient, and who lets the patient know what his plans for treatment are, will find that the patient appreciates and responds to this respectful attitude. When sessions with other family members are held, the patient should be present whenever feasible. This can reduce the likelihood that he will feel the therapist and his family are doing things behind his back.

A similar flexibility and willingness to place the patient's interests foremost is a sound guideline for any decision that may arise in psychotherapy. The patient who feels he is being treated as an adult by a physician who appeals to the intact and healthy part of his personality, will often respond by taking appropriate control of some of his previously disorganized behavior. Most patients can cooperate to a large degree even in a decision such as entering a psychiatric hospital.

In summary, while medications are usually indispensable in treating the psychosis per se, psychotherapy involves treating the patient as a whole person, discovering and fostering the patient's own abilities to control his behavior and to resume competent social functioning. The human context of the patient–physician relationship is important to the patient, for in this collaborative effort he will be learning the necessary tool of clear communication with another person.

Working with the family remains an important consideration in treatment of schizophrenic patients, also.

The patient's family is often a potential and necessary ally. Families can be extremely helpful in carrying out diagnostic evaluation and treatment; they can provide information the patient may be unable to give, and a session with all the family can often demonstrate to the physician much about the ways the family deals with problems and stress. He can then counsel the family on using certain approaches to the patient and avoiding other behavior that places undue pressures or demands on the patient.

In addition, if the patient is out of the hospital for most of his treatment, the family can help supervise his taking medication, getting to clinic or office appointments, and other necessary treatment activities. If the patient is hospitalized, close planning among the hospital staff, the patient, his family, and the people who will be responsible for afterhospital care is essential to provide a smooth transition back to home and the community.

SOCIAL THERAPY

Social therapy is the term applied to treatment approaches that affect social functioning and behavior of patients. These approaches include inpatient hospital care, aftercare programs, and vocational/educational rehabilitation. All of these treatment modalities have some place in the planning of each patient's treatment; they should be applied with the same deliberate care that one uses in prescribing a particular dose of a certain medication at a certain point in an illness. Like medications, social therapies can be efficacious when used as indicated, and like medications social therapies can have undesirable effects when used indiscriminately.

Hospitalization is an important tool in psychiatric treatment. Intensive supervision can literally enable a patient to survive a suicidal crisis or a period of irrational excitement and overactivity. Planned therapeutic programs during a hospital stay can allow a patient to discover his abilities and assets, and to find ways to use them to lead a more stable life. The shelter or asylum provided in any hospital stay can be an opportunity to take stock, to sort out the various forces and demands in one's life, and to make plans to deal effectively with these stresses rather than becoming overwhelmed by them. Living together with other people in a unit of an inpatient service can be a new experience in sharing and developing human relationships, something that schizophrenic patients often have great difficulty doing on their own.

There are several relative indications for hospitalizing a patient, and a few conditions for which hospitalization is absolutely necessary. The absolute indications include severe suicidal risk, profound withdrawal or excitement in a catatonic state, and extreme disorganization that makes it impossible for a patient to cooperate in controlling his own behavior. In situations less severe than these, the decision for hospitalization is made by balancing the benefits of hospital care; the patient's relative ability to cooperate and participate in his own treatment; the available alternatives such as daily office or clinic visits, partial hospital services (day hospital), the ability of family to help supervise the patient; and the possible risks of hospital care (eg, increased inappropriate dependency; loss of social role, such as job).

A patient who requires close supervision because of a rapidly changing clinical state, who presents a problem in diagnosis, or who requires large doses of a medication not taken before, may receive better care if he is hospitalized during the initial stage of treatment. Likewise, the patient who has a disrupted life with little or no family or other social support may require hospitalization for effective treatment.

Chronically ill schizophrenic patients may be hospitalized briefly and periodically when their families need a respite from the full responsibility of caring for them. These respite hospitalizations can be an opportunity for patient, family, and physician to reevaluate the total approach to long-term treatment. Such a hospitalization is generally time-limited, and discharge is planned from the day of admission.

Facilities for inpatient psychiatric care vary from community to community. The several types are psychiatric beds or units in a general hospital, private psychiatric hospitals, and public (state or county) psychiatric hospitals. General hospital psychiatric services have increased greatly in the last 20 years, and such inpatient units can offer intensive diagnostic and therapeutic care during a short-term hospitalization. Care in such general hospital units is usually covered by Blue Cross and other medical insurance policies. Another advantage of the general hospital psychiatric unit is that it is usually close to the patient's home and family, so a smooth transition can be made at discharge.

Private psychiatric hospitals offer long-term care, generally, and can provide intensive therapy for patients who may require several months of inpatient care to regain function. They often have specialized units or specific psychiatrists who have concentrated on doing therapy with difficult schizophrenic patients.

State and county public psychiatric hospitals offer both acute and chronic care. For a patient who has no medical insurance, a brief hospitalization in a public hospital may be the only choice if he is too ill for outpatient care. State hospitals have changed over the years also, and many patients are discharged within a few weeks, to return to community-based outpatient care. The patient who has not responded to therapy, and who cannot live independently or with family in the community, may require indefinitely long inpatient care. Here the state hospital may be the place of choice for those with limited or exhausted financial means.

Most patients will agree to voluntary hospital care, but some will refuse or be unable to cooperate. In these instances, the physician must decide if he will begin commitment procedures to require the patient to enter a hospital involuntarily. Different states have different regulations about involuntary admission; a usual situation for which involuntary admission is allowable is the patient who, because of his psychiatric illness, presents an immediate danger to himself (suicide; risk-taking, such as running into traffic) or to others (threats of assault or homicide). In most states two physicians examine the patient, and if they both find that he is psychiatrically ill and presents a danger, they sign the appropriate papers. These papers are then presented to the receiving hospital, by family or by the court system. Involuntarily admitted patients are examined, treated, and subsequently their situation is reviewed to determine if they still require involuntary hospitalization. Virtually all public mental hospitals receive involuntary patients, and many private psychiatric hospitals also do so.

After hospitalization some patients return to their homes, while others are referred to a halfway house for further therapy in a setting where they can take some steps toward independence, within a structured and planned environment. Halfway houses, in which patients generally stay three to ten months, are located within communities, and patients living there often take part-time or full-time jobs, or return to school. In these facilities patients can further develop social abilities and at the same time keep a distance from some of the family tensions and demands that may have exacerbated their illness.

Whether a patient goes home, or to a halfway house, or lives on his own after hospitalization, a well-planned aftercare program is an essential step in ensuring maximum opportunity for recovery. This can be done within the same institution that provided the inpatient care, or by another outpatient clinic, or by a private practitioner with the collaboration of social or rehabilitation services. A particularly useful model of aftercare is described by Donlon and Rada.[6] It includes group therapy of a supportive nature, medications, socialization groups in which patients can further develop their social skills, and aggressive follow-up for any patient who misses an appointment. Patients become loyal to such an aftercare program, and can readily turn to it for as much as they may need in any stage of their recovery. At the same time, a good aftercare program will place definite demands upon its patients, challenging them in a supportive fashion to make the most of their lives by seeking jobs or education.

Vocational and educational rehabilitation services can help many recovering patients to return to former occupations or to choose new fields better suited to their abilities and their vulnerabilities. These services, usually run by state or local departments of education, can also provide some financial support for patients in the transition from dependent hospital patient to productive member of the community. A further note here: a trend in state laws is to forbid employers to refuse a job to someone merely because the person has been a mental patient. Therefore, when the general job market is good, the prospects of a patient finding a job may also be good; every effort should be made to help a recovering patient gain the necessary skills to obtain employment.

Other therapies should be briefly mentioned. Electroconvulsive therapy, used mostly for psychotic depressions, also may provide quicker recovery than would medications for a schizophrenic patient in a catatonic withdrawal. Megavitamin therapy, with high doses of nicotinic acid and other vitamins, has not been shown to offer any significant help for schizophrenic patients; in fact, most reports of the treatment include large groups of patients who have been given phenothiazines in addition to the vitamins, and results are equivocal at best.

In summary then, there are effective therapeutic approaches for patients with schizophrenic illnesses. It is a matter of finding the combination of approaches that best fits the individual patient. Antipsychotic medication, some form of psychotherapy, and a plan to improve social functioning are all essential components. Most patients can gain significant improvement, and many will recover completely. Lehmann states that

of patients hospitalized for an acute schizophrenic episode, 60 percent
will show good social recovery in a five-year follow-up, 30 percent will
have some handicaps, and only 10 percent will be in a hospital.[9]

REFERENCES

1. Arieti S: An overview of schizophrenia from a predominately psychological
   approach. Am J Psychiatry 131:241, 1974
2. Ayd FJ: Depot fluphenazines. Reappraisal of 10 years' clinical experience.
   Am J Psychiatry 132:491, 1975
3. Babigian HM: Schizophrenia. Etiology. In Freedman AM, Kaplan HI,
   Sadock BJ (eds): Comprehensive Textbook of Psychiatry, 2nd ed. Baltimore,
   Williams and Wilkins, 1975
4. Bleuler M: Conception of schizophrenia within the last fifty years. Int J
   Psychiatry 1:501, 1965
5. Cancro R: Some diagnostic and therapeutic considerations on the schizophrenic syndrome. Psychiatry Digest 37:13, 1976
6. Donlon PT, Rada RT: Issues in developing quality aftercare clinics for the
   chronic mentally ill. Community Ment Health J 12:29, 1976
7. Kety SD, Rosenthal P, Wender F, et al: Mental illness in the biological and
   adoptive families of adopted individuals who have become schizophrenic. A
   preliminary report based on psychiatric interviews. In Fieve R, Rosenthal D,
   Brill H (eds): Genetic Research in Psychiatry. Baltimore, Johns Hopkins
   Univ Press, 1975
8. Klein DF, Davis JM: Diagnosis and Drug Treatment of Psychiatric Disorders. Baltimore, Williams and Wilkins, 1969
9. Lehmann H: Schizophrenia. Clinical features. In Freedman AM, Kaplan HI,
   Sadock BJ (eds): Comprehensive Textbook of Psychiatry, 2nd ed. Baltimore,
   Williams and Wilkins, 1975
10. Oppenheimer H: Clinical Psychiatry. New York, Harper & Row, 1971
11. Snyder SH: The dopamine hypothesis of schizophrenia. Focus on the
    dopamine receptor. Am J Psychiatry 133:197, 1976
12. Stephens JH: Long-term course and prognosis in schizophrenia. Semin
    Psychiatry 2:464, 1970

PART
IV

EVALUATION AND
MANAGEMENT

Chapter

16

Psychiatric Evaluation of the Medical Patient

Psychiatric evaluation closely resembles the rest of medical evaluation in its goals and methods.

The ultimate goal of the psychiatric evaluation is to establish a comprehensive diagnosis which can lead to an effective plan of management.[2] Comprehensive psychiatric diagnosis includes several components, which will be described below.

Methods of psychiatric evaluation consist of history taking, examination of the patient's mental functioning, and the interpretation of appropriate special tests or procedures. Most information comes through the interview with the patient, and the principles and techniques of this essential procedure will be discussed in detail.

One must decide how extensive the psychiatric evaluation should be for a particular patient. Several factors enter into this including presentation of evidence suggesting psychiatric conditions, the probable diagnosis, and the severity and urgency of the patient's problems. In addition, the primary physician will generally conduct a more extensive psychiatric evaluation when he plans to assume continuing responsibility for clinical management, with or without psychiatric consultation; if he plans to refer the patient to a psychiatrist for management of the psychiatric problems, he may do a briefer psychiatric evaluation. Decisions regarding continuing management of the patient can of course be made after consultation; such variables as those already mentioned (probable diagnosis, severity and urgency of the patient's condition) will enter into this decision of who should manage the patient. The indications for psychiatric referral and the importance of making the referral in such a way as to facilitate acceptance and to minimize the likelihood of the patient's feeling misunderstood or rejected are discussed in Chapter 17.

GOALS

Comprehensive psychiatric diagnosis includes (1) delineation of symptomatic and functional problems, (2) identification of a psychiatric syndrome or disorder, (3) assessment of factors which contribute to etiology, and (4) assessment of personal assets and resources.

DELINEATION OF PROBLEMS

By psychiatric problems we refer to symptomatic complaints and difficulties in functioning, or behavior which stems from mental or emotional disturbance. Psychiatric problems may be related to (1) difficulties in cognition such as disorientation, poor memory, delusions, concretistic thinking, and hallucinations; (2) disturbance of feeling or mood such as depression, elation, and anxiety; (3) disordered function and somatic complaints (without discernible organic basis) such as insomnia, fatigue, anorexia, impotence, and headache; and (4) patterns of maladaptive behavior such as repeated inability to get along with persons in authority. Occasionally, patients will consult the primary physician because of a difficulty in their present life situation. Of the aforementioned types of problems, probably the most commonly encountered presenting complaint seen by the primary physician is that of functional or somatic symptoms without organic basis. It is wise to keep in mind that occasionally a patient may use a physical symptom that has an organic cause as an admission ticket to see the physician about an emotional problem.

Frequently, in the course of the clinical investigation, a group of problems emerges as a recognizable clinical entity or psychiatric disorder. When this occurs, definitive treatment is aimed at alleviation of the disorder, such as depression, with the reasonable expectation that relief from associated problems such as insomnia, anorexia, or loss of sexual interest will be obtained as the depression improves. However, as crucial as treatment of the underlying disorder is, the management of symptomatic manifestations or problems is also important and sometimes must be initiated before a comprehensive diagnosis is established.

For example, the physician, upon discerning that the patient presents evidence of emotional disturbance, must decide whether the disturbance constitutes an emergency. If an emergency exists, a preliminary management plan must be instituted without delay even though comprehensive diagnosis is not yet established. Psychiatric emergencies are discussed in Chapter 7. Here it may simply be noted that a psychiatric emergency exists when the patient is experiencing acute, intense suffering requiring immediate attention or when his behavior, actual or potential, is alarming. Probably the most common example of the latter is seen in the patient who poses a serious suicidal risk.

In addition to emergency situations, there are many psychiatric problems which warrant specific management in addition to longer range, definitive treatment of the underlying disorder. Severe insomnia, for example, may not only be a symptom of depression (or some other condition) but may itself significantly contribute to the patient's feeling of fatigue and apprehension; for this reason, the physician may attempt to provide the depressed patient relief from this symptom while awaiting the patient's response to antidepressant medication. Similarly, the confusion and panic of delirium pose problems that require careful management while determination and treatment of the underlying causes of the condition are underway. Severe anorexia or refusal to eat calls for careful monitoring of the patient's nutritional status regardless of the underlying disorder.

PSYCHIATRIC DISORDERS

Psychiatric illness can be defined as being any condition in which there is suffering and disability resulting primarily from a disorder of thinking, feeling, or behavior. This definition clearly encompasses (1) the organic brain syndromes, (2) the psychoses, (3) the neuroses, (4) the psychophysiologic disorders, (5) painful or disabling situational disturbances, (6) alcoholism, and (7) drug dependence. There has been considerable disagreement about the inclusion of personality disorders in the general rubric of psychiatric illness. However, there is little doubt that in some instances the enduring maladaptive attitudes and behavior of personality disorders do result in disability and suffering.

Table 1 gives a classification of the major psychiatric disorders; each (with the exception of mental retardation) is discussed elsewhere. Here we will only briefly describe some of the salient features which are useful in differentiating between several of the major categories of psychiatric illness. In arriving at a diagnosis, the clinician will find it practical to approach diagnostic categorization by proceeding from the broad categories to more restricted ones, and finally to specific entities.

The first categorization is to distinguish organic disorders from functional disorders. Here the clinician must be alert not only to evidences of

---

Table 1. Classification of Psychiatric Disorders

1. Mental Retardation
2. Disorders Associated with Organic Impairment of Cerebral Function
   A. Organic brain syndromes
   B. Organic conditions in which the characteristic features of OBS are absent, eg, psychosis associated with amphetamine intoxication
3. Psychoses without Presently Known Organic Impairment of Cerebral Function
   A. Schizophrenic disorders
   B. Major affective disorders
      Unipolar manic illness
      Depressive illness
      a. Primary
         Unipolar
         Bipolar
      b. Secondary
4. Neuroses
5. Personality Disorders
6. Sexual Disorders
7. Alcoholism and Drug Dependence
8. Psychophysiologic Disturbances
9. Transient Situational Disturbances

---

the organic brain syndromes but also to organic diseases, such as hyperthyroidism, which can simulate emotional disorders. Organic brain syndromes (OBS) are characterized by impairment of orientation, memory, judgment, and other intellectual functions, such as comprehension and calculation; lability and shallowness of affect are often present. Nevertheless, psychoses caused by toxic substances are not invariably accompanied by these classic symptoms of OBS; a notable example is the psychosis associated with amphetamine intoxication which closely resembles acute paranoid schizophrenia and in which the sensorium is usually clear.

If organic causes seem unlikely, the next step is to distinguish between the functional psychoses (schizophrenia and affective disorders) and the nonpsychotic disorders (neuroses, personality disorders, and situational reactions). The term functional psychoses refers to those disorders which, in fully developed form, gravely impair mental functioning, grossly interfere with the patient's ability to cope with the ordinary demands of life, and for which, at the present time, no physical etiology has been definitely identified. The two main categories of functional psychoses are the schizophrenic disorders and the major affective disorders.

Schizophrenia includes a group of disorders manifested by misinterpretation of reality, interference with thought associations (blocking, concrete thinking, etc), delusions, hallucinations, marked ambivalence, flatness or inappropriateness of affect, withdrawal, and regressive or bizarre behavior; the sensorium is clear. The major affective disorders are characterized by depression or mania or, alternatingly, both. Depression is characterized by feelings of sadness, guilt, and hopelessness, decrease in interest in and ability to experience pleasure, attitudes of self-deprecation and pessimism, fatigue, psychomotor retardation, insomnia, poor appetite, weight loss, and a variety of somatic symptoms. Mania is characterized by an elated mood or irritability, hypertalkativeness, and hyperactivity. In schizophrenia and the affective disorders, the severity and variety of symptoms are reduced considerably during the incipient stage or convalescent stage of the illness; at these stages, or in other less than fully developed forms of the disorder, the illness may not have reached psychotic proportions.

The neuroses are characterized by (1) symptoms of anxiety such as fear, tenseness, palpitations, and sweaty palms; (2) symptoms which serve partially to alleviate or localize anxiety such as phobias, obsessions, compulsions, hypochondriasis, and conversion; or (3) both overt anxiety and anxiety-related symptoms. There is no evidence of disorientation or other impairment of intellectual function, nor is there evidence of distortions of reality recognition or of perception, and the patient is usually clearly aware that he has an emotional or psychologic disturbance.

Psychophysiologic disorders are characterized by physical symptoms accompanying physiologic changes produced by emotional factors. The hyperventilation syndrome is an example.

Alcoholism and drug dependence refer to conditions in which alcohol or drug consumption is damaging to physical health, interferes with personal and social functioning, or is associated with psychologic or physical dependence.

Situational disturbances refer to disorders which develop as a response to severe environmental stress and which abate when the stress is removed. This diagnosis is usually reserved for persons in whom there is no evidence of preexisting mental or emotional disorder.

Personality disorders are characterized by deeply ingrained maladaptive attitudes and patterns of behavior which often become manifest in adolescence or earlier; there is relatively little evidence of overt anxiety or other neurotic symptoms.

It is apparent that these categories of illness are not mutually exclusive. Patients with schizophrenic illness, depression, neurosis, or personality disorder may become dependent upon drugs or alcohol and are not immune to the development of organic brain syndromes. Organic disease affecting cerebral function may precipitate a depression, severe anxiety, or paranoid delusions, or may exacerbate an already existing emotional disorder.

ASSESSMENT OF ETIOLOGIC FACTORS

Modern medical practitioners have long desired to aim treatment at the cause or causes of illness and not to rest content with symptom alleviation alone. Further, it has become increasingly apparent that the concept of a simple one-to-one relationship between a single cause and a single effect (disease) does not apply to most types of illness; clearly, it does not apply to psychiatric disorders. In considering the etiology of psychiatric disorders it is helpful to bear two concepts in mind: (1) most (perhaps all) psychiatric disorders result from the convergence of more than one etiologic factor; and (2) psychiatric disorders unfold in an epigenetic manner, ie, what has already developed partially determines what is to be developed. Thus, the clinician is interested in ascertaining those factors which were present at the time of onset or exacerbation of the illness, in understanding the epigenetic sequence of illness development, and, where possible, in applying his grasp of etiology to the planning of treatment and management.

The process of diagnostic categorization discussed above yields some knowledge of etiology and serves to direct the clinican along certain lines of investigation. This is clearly the case, for example, when the intermediate diagnosis is organic brain syndrome or when, even in the absence of the usual symptoms of OBS, the clinican suspects that a physical or toxic factor is present; the physician then begins a systematic inquiry into the possibilities with particular emphasis on the discernment of those contributory factors which can be removed or modified by treatment. In this example, the aim of the investigation is to narrow the diagnosis to an etiologically specific type of OBS, such as toxic psychosis secondary to barbiturate withdrawal, and then to plan management accordingly.

In the example of toxic psychosis secondary to barbiturate withdrawal, the immediate precipitating event is, of course, the cessation of barbiturate ingestion. The epigenetic sequence which preceded the toxic psychosis includes (1) those psychologic, social, and other factors which led the patient to "need" or want hypnotic drugs; and (2) the actual ingestion of barbiturates in sufficient amount and for a sufficient period of time to establish physical dependence. Obviously, the investigation of the factors which contributed to the establishment of the addiction requires the collaboration of the patient (and often his family), and is crucial to the planning of long-range treatment aimed at assisting the patient with underlying emotional problems and at preventing a recurrence of the addiction.

The contributory factors in emotional disorders include (1) hereditary predisposition; (2) preillness personality development and adaptation; (3) life situation around the onset, remission, and exacerbation of illness episodes; and (4) present life situation.

For example, the clinician may learn that the depressive illness of a middle-aged woman began around the time her youngest child married and left home (the "empty-nest syndrome"). The physician knows that most women do not become clinically depressed by such an event in their lives. What is there about the patient that apparently predisposed her to react to that event with depression? A number of contributory factors might be ascertained upon further investigation. Not uncommonly it is learned that the patient has long led a rather narrow, constricted life, deriving her feeling of worthwhileness almost entirely from her role as mother, and that a certain distance between the patient and her husband has slowly developed over a period of years. In this setting, the departure of her youngest child has left the patient feeling virtually roleless and unneeded. The patient may or may not require an antidepressant medicine but, in any event, drug treatment alone is doomed to failure in the long run, for she will require support, thoughtful assistance, and perhaps the cooperation of her spouse in order to develop new roles for herself, necessary to the restoration and maintenance of her self-esteem.

PERSONAL ASSETS AND RESOURCES

Physicians generally tend to focus much of their attention on pathology, on "what is wrong" with their patients. This is hardly surprising in view of the fact that, in the overwhelming majority of instances, patients visit physicians only when they are having troubles of one kind or another.

Nonetheless, the physician utilizes and engages that part of the patient which is healthy when he undertakes treatment of any condition, although he may do this more or less automatically or unconsciously. In our view, it is just as advisable deliberately to assess the areas of psychologic health and other assets of the patient when the physician is dealing with a person who is emotionally ill, as it is to assess cardiopulmonary function prior to surgery. In setting therapeutic goals, it is helpful to know how well the patient was getting along in the various areas of his life prior to the present illness.

At a very elementary level, the physician obviously must have some notion of the patient's general level of intelligence, mastery of the language, and memory, for without this he will not know if the patient is able to comprehend and cooperate with the plan of treatment. Less obvious, but equally important, are the patient's desire to get well, his ability to place trust in the physician and others, his ability to make relevant observations about himself and others, and his willingness to report these observations to his physician.

Often, in the course of treatment of emotional illness, the patient's values, goals, and commitments to significant other people in his life become key foundation stones on which recovery is constructed. In this connection, it is noteworthy that sometimes an attitude or value system which was implicated in the genesis of emotional illness may also be utilized in recovery from it. The empty-nest–syndrome patient mentioned previously, who had too narrowly based her raison d'être on the care of her children, obviously places great value on relating to people who need her. This fact can be put to use in reviewing the marital relationship with both the patient and her husband, and in helping the patient to seek opportunities for the personal gratification of "being needed" outside the home; further, it may be useful tactfully to explore with the patient the possibility that in her zeal to be a good mother she unwittingly may have made it difficult for others to reciprocate, and thus may have contributed to the distance between herself and her husband.

Family, social, and financial resources must also be evaluated in order for them to be utilized therapeutically and to avoid imposing upon the patient a plan of care which is impossible to carry out.

METHODS

The principal method of psychiatric evaluation consists of history taking and mental status examination by means of interviewing the patient.[3,5,6] Interviewing includes observations of the patient's behavior and verbal exchanges that occur during the physical examination. In addition to the interview, the physician may arrange for the administration and interpretation of special tests or procedures if these are required to complete the examination in selected cases.[14]

THE PSYCHIATRIC INTERVIEW

In conducting the interview, the physician is in the roles of both participant and observer.[5,6] In practice, these two activities of participation and observation are so interrelated as to be virtually inseparable.

What the physician observes or otherwise learns about the patient as the interview proceeds influences his approach to the patient and the particular areas of inquiry he chooses to emphasize. A particular historic item or observation stimulates a train of associations in the physician's mind which may in turn lead him to make specific inquiries to test a hypothesis. For example, anorexia or refusal to eat in an adolescent female brings to mind the possibility of anorexia nervosa; in a guarded suspicious person, the possibility of a paranoid delusion of food being poisoned; in a histrionic, seductive person, the possibility of a neurotic basis with the appetite loss being used to manipulate someone; in a person of any age, but particularly middle age and older, the possibility of depression. Various physical possibilities, such as hepatitis or carcinoma of the colon or pancreas, may also occur to the interviewer even when the anorexia appears to be part of a depressive syndrome. The interviewer may elect to postpone the pursuit of a particular hypothesis until some later point in the interview, if in his judgment the patient's spontaneous speech is currently centered upon other relevant topics or on issues which are important to the patient (and therefore also to the interviewer); the physician will also postpone a particular line of inquiry if he feels that the patient's sensitivity or defensiveness makes such a course wise for the time being.

In addition, the interviewer's attitudes, manner, and phraseology affect how the patient feels and therefore influence what he chooses to reveal verbally and in nonverbal behavior.

Principles and Techniques   To gain the most information from the patient and to be of the most help, the clinician must arrange a setting in which the patient is at ease and is assured of the interviewer's complete attention. Privacy must be assured, when possible, by a separate room; a busy public ward is paradoxically more private than is a shared double room. Interruptions destroy the continuity of the patient's story and his sense that the clinician deems this story important. Therefore, phone calls, paging, and other disturbances should be held or delayed. A certain length of time is also necessary to establish a working relationship. An hour is generally necessary to conduct a full psychiatric interview. To ensure hearing the patient's story rather than what the patient thinks the examiner wants to hear, one should maintain a free-ranging approach, beginning with what the patient is most ready to tell. Open-ended questions instead of those which can be answered "Yes" or "No" yield more complete information.

The interviewer strives to establish rapport with the patient. His effort is frequently complicated by the fact that patients with emotional problems or illnesses often tend to suffer from loss of self-esteem. This, in part, stems from the patient's notion that mental illness itself indicates personal failure or inadequacy. Further, the illness is sometimes the surface manifestation of underlying problems and conflicts which are associated with painful feelings that are partially allayed, avoided, and revealed by specific symptoms. Therefore, in developing rapport with the patient, the physician needs to be mindful of these two related issues of self-esteem and defensiveness.

SELF-ESTEEM. The interviewer proceeds in a manner that conveys respect, interest, and, if possible, intellectual and empathic understanding. He conducts the interview with an attitude that he and the patient are engaged in a collaborative undertaking which has as its goal (1) a better understanding of the patient's problems, (2) an understanding of the patient himself, and (3) assistance in returning him to a state of well-being. The deliberate adoption of this attitude carries the message that the patient's role is an active one in which he works with the physician and not a merely passive one of receiving advice and pills.

Not uncommonly, a distressed person who is seeking help will tend to idealize the physician, perceiving him as a person of exceptional wisdom, knowledge, understanding, and skill. This idealization is often manifest even though the patient has had virtually no experience with the physician. This in part stems from the patient's need to feel confidence and trust in his doctor. As the patient gains more experience wih the physician, this initial, illusory idealization is gradually replaced by a more realistically based appraisal of the physician's reliability, competence, and therapeutic intent.

DEFENSES One of the most common defenses encountered by the general physician is that of somatization, in which the patient simultaneously avoids and reveals emotional problems by focusing on one or more physical complaints. The depressed patient, for example, may complain of fatigue or of some bodily pain for which no organic basis can be found. He may tend to minimize feelings of depression or dismiss such feelings as secondary to one or another physical symptom.

It is a useful technique to respect the patient's somatization of his problems by encouraging him to recount fully his complaints and their chronologic development. During this phase of the interview, the physician listens for spontaneous references to feelings and experiences which may provide openings for inquiry into personal and emotional issues that are related to the problems underlying the somatic defenses. In proceeding in this fashion, the interviewer is taking advantage of the patient's associative processes to get clues to feelings, fantasies, and experiences relevant to the present illness. If the pursuit of a given line of inquiry arouses discomfort, the patient may temporarily return to somatic symptoms or some other psychologically safe area. The physician should be attuned to these defensive shifts in the conversation, for they enable the interviewer to develop hypotheses about what may be troubling the patient. These may be confirmed or refuted as he gets more data.[2,5]

It is often revealing to ask the patient for his own theories about what is causing his physical (or other) complaints, and to elicit from him the consequences of his somatic symptoms. The usefulness of the latter inquiry was exemplified by a patient who explained that the numbness and weakness of her hands, for which no organic basis could be found, would make it impossible for her to hold and otherwise care for a baby. It was learned that the patient wanted out of her marriage and that her physical symptoms developed a day or two after she first suspected that she was pregnant.

TACT   In conducting the mental status examination, the interviewer includes an assessment of intellectual functions such as memory, concentration, and orientation. In carrying out this part of the interview, it is important to be aware that most people are uncomfortable if they feel their mental functioning is being tested. It is, therefore, helpful to soften the impact of an otherwise jarring question by tactfully giving it a rationale in the context of the interview. For example, one may comment to the patient that, in view of certain symptoms or problems with which he has been suffering, it would seem likely that he has been preoccupied and perhaps has found it difficult to concentrate and keep track of the details of daily life. This can be followed by stating that the examiner would, therefore, like to ask several questions which will help him to assess these aspects of the patient's functioning.

VERBAL AND NONVERBAL BEHAVIOR   During the interview, the physician is interested not only in what the patient says but in how he says it: the structure or form of his speech and accompanying affect as well as its content. He will also take note of topics which the patient completely avoids or, as mentioned previously, those which prompt the patient to change the subject. The interviewer will also observe nonverbal aspects of behavior as revealed in facial expression, gestures, and posture, or as implied by the patient's general appearance, including neatness, appropriateness of attire, and nutritional status.

COLLATERAL INTERVIEWS

It is often advisable to interview one or more members of the patient's family or, occasionally, a friend of the patient. This is particularly the case when the patient's illness has seriously impaired his ability to give historic data that are important in diagnosis, or when the cooperation of the family is necessary in order to proceed with further evaluation or treatment. In addition, the patient's emotional difficulties may be so intertwined with the attitudes and behavior of key members of the family that the interviewer must include family members in the evaluation in order to achieve comprehensive diagnosis and to plan treatment. Collateral interviews are, in a way, the psychiatric equivalent of laboratory examinations, since they can yield new information from a different source.

As a general rule, it is strongly advisable to interview relatives or other interested persons only after the reasons for doing so have been discussed with the patient and his consent obtained. Rarely, an exception to this must be made, as with an acutely psychotic or self-destructive patient who does not give the physician permission to talk with responsible next of kin.

Sometimes, a well-intentioned relative will offer to give the physician information about the patient with the provision that the physician keep the information or the source of it secret. When this occurs, the physician should explain that such information would be useless to him unless he is at liberty to use his own discretion about discussing the information with the patient and revealing its source. In the great majority of instances, the relative sees the sense in this policy and withdraws his insistence upon secrecy. The physician should, in most situations, freely discuss with the patient the content of interviews with other informants. In fact, it is often quite appropriate to invite the patient to be present and to participate when relatives or others are interviewed.

PHYSICAL EXAMINATION

The general physical and neurologic examinations afford the clinician an excellent opportunity to make observations and inquiries relevant to the patient's emotional or mental condition. For example, observations of weight loss, fine tremor, moist palms, constricted pupils, dilated pupils, or skin excoriations provide important clues to further investigation.

PSYCHOLOGIC TESTING

Psychologic testing is a valuable adjunct to the psychiatric examination in several circumstances.[1,4]

1. Determination of intelligence level. This may be useful in cases of school failure, apparent inadequacy at work, or when one suspects that the patient is seriously underchallenged by his occupation.
2. Psychologic testing may be helpful when the clinical picture is equivocal. For example, standardized tests of higher cerebral function are useful when one suspects organic brain damage resulting in changes too slight or subtle to be detected by the conventional mental status examination.
3. Certain psychologic tests may reveal psychodynamic themes or personality traits which were not discerned clearly during the interview.
4. Symptom inventories and other types of clinical "scales" are sometimes used to establish a quantitative estimate of the patient's illness or symptomatic status, and may be repeated one or more times in order to observe the effect of therapeutic intervention.

There are a variety of psychologic tests available. Some, such as the Rorschach, Wechsler Adult Intelligence Scale, and the Thematic Apperception Test, are administered by trained psychologists. Others, such as the Minnesota Multiphasic Personality Inventory and a variety of clinical "scales" to assess symptomatic states, are self-administered but are scored by the physician or the psychologist.

SPECIAL DIAGNOSTIC PROCEDURES

It is apparent that thorough psychiatric evaluation of the patient cannot be separated from the total medical evaluation. It would be folly, for example, to assume that a particular somatic complaint is without an organic basis because the patient happens to be depressed or because the symptom appeared at a time when the patient was experiencing emotional stress. While it is true that the physician cannot prove a negative, ie, that organic disease is absent, it is also true that both he and the patient need to be assured that all reasonable diagnostic tests for physical illness have been done. What constitutes "reasonable" depends upon the physician's judgment in a particular clinical situation. There is no quicker way to alienate a patient than by giving him the impression that his complaints have not been taken seriously or that the physician jumped to the conclusion that they are "psychologic."

Because of the frequency with which emotionally disturbed patients have symptoms referable to the nervous system (headaches, giddiness, tremor, weakness, tingling sensations, difficulties in concentrating, etc), careful neurologic evaluation is always indicated and may, in selected cases, include neurologic consultations and special diagnostic studies such as an electroencephalogram, skull x-ray, or more elaborate procedures.

Specific steps useful in confirming the diagnosis of addiction to hypnotic drugs and opiates are discussed in Chapter 10.

CONTINUED OBSERVATIONS

More often than not, thorough evaluation and comprehension of the patient's problems require a number of contacts over a period of time. Occasionally, a brief period of hospitalization, in which the patient can be observed by a trained staff, is necessary for adequate diagnostic evaluation.

ORGANIZATION OF DATA

Although the actual order in which data are collected depends upon a number of factors, the clinician should have a mental outline of key areas of the history and the present mental status that are to be covered in carrying out a psychiatric evaluation.

HISTORY

The organization of historic information does not differ essentially from that usually obtained in general medical evaluation of the patient. In the case of psychiatric illness, somewhat more emphasis is placed upon a detailed psychosocial history because this is often crucial to understanding the development of the presenting problem, the present illness, previous episodes of illness and remissions from illness, the preillness level of adaptation, and the patient's personality and development. It is useful to organize psychosocial data temporally and topically.

Temporally, psychosocial data can be organized as follows: (1) present life situation; (2) life situation concurrent with the present illness; (3) in the case of previous episodes of illness, life situation concurrent with onset of the first episode of illness and its remission; and (4) psychosocial history prior to the illness. The interviewer is particularly interested in events or circumstances in the patient's life, such as those involving family, friends, and work, which may have contributed to emotional disturbances, which may be secondary to maladaptive behavior, or which may be indicative of resources and strengths potentially useful in management and recovery.

Within these temporal groups, psychosocial data can be further organized topically. The major topics to be covered are included in the history outline given below.

OUTLINE OF HISTORY

1. *Identifying Data*. Name, age, sex, race, marital status, and occupation.

2. *Presenting Problems*. These should be recorded in the patient's own words.
3. *Present Illness*. This consists of a detailed chronologic reconstruction of the present illness (or present episode of illness) from its inception to the present. While obtaining the present illness history, it is important to ascertain why the patient decided to consult the physician at this time. This is particularly relevant if the presenting problems have existed for some time. It is important to know if the patient seeks help because of his own concern or at the behest of some other person or agency; did he select the physician or was he referred by someone?

   In the case of psychiatric illness, it is not uncommon for the patient to report aspects of his life situation that are temporally associated with features of the illness. He may or may not regard these aspects of his life situation as causally related to his problems but the fact that they are associatively linked to his problems is worthy of note.
4. *Past Psychiatric History*. Previous episodes of psychiatric illness similar to or different from the present illness are noted. Approximate dates of onsets and remissions should be recorded as these may be of significance when a chronologically parallel psychosocial history is obtained; type of treatment obtained for previous illnesses also gives clues in planning management.

   Has the patient had a history of mood swings, history of symptoms suggestive of episodes of anxiety or of chronic tension, phobias, obsessions, compulsions, somatic symptoms suggestive of conversion hysteria, and other symptoms indicative of neurosis; psychophysiologic symptoms; maladaptive patterns of recent change in attitudes or customary ways of behaving?
5. *Past Medical History*. This includes any history of significant illnesses, surgical procedures, accidents, injuries, and review of systems.
6. *History of Alcohol and Drug Intake*. The amount, type of substance, regularity and duration of use, and route of administration are recorded. A patient's defensiveness may pose a barrier to obtaining an accurate history; this may be reduced if one begins by inquiring about the more acceptable substances such as coffee and tobacco. In addition, one can engage the patient's interest and often form judgments about the actual amounts consumed by inquiring about the effects the patient experiences from his use of substances.
7. *Present Household and Family History*. It is often convenient to initiate inquiry into this area by asking the patient to name persons who presently live in his home and their kinship or relationship to him. This inquiry usually provides a natural opening for obtaining information about the patient's spouse, his children, and other relatives who are involved in the patient's current and past life, including parents and siblings.

It is particularly important to obtain the patient's description of the personalities of the important people in his current family or household and the family of origin, and his relationship with them. The interviewer is particularly alert to important or disturbing events in the patient's family life which are temporally associated with illnesses in the present or past; this includes events such as marital separation, divorce, departure of children from the home, illnesses, and deaths. The incidence of psychiatric or other illness in the family not only provides data relevant to hereditary predisposition, but may also provide a clue about the patient's fears regarding the health of himself or his children.

8. *Occupation and Economic Status*. This includes the type of work in which the patient is engaged, job satisfaction, relationship with peers and supervisors at present and in the past. Patient's assessment of financial condition, eg, adequacy of income in relation to needs, indebtedness, is also noted. Does work history suggest that the patient tends to move upward when he changes jobs, or that he shifts from one job to another because of difficulties at work? Has he persisted in his present work situation because he likes his work or because it offers him security or both? Is the patient approaching retirement? If so, what are his feelings about it?

9. *Recent Psychosexual History*. This includes the patient's sexual preferences; the quality or degree of satisfaction in the sexual relationship with spouse; problems in functioning, such as decline of sexual interest, impotence, premature ejaculation, retarded ejaculation, anorgasmia, and dyspareunia; concern about homosexual feelings or behavior; and history of sexual affairs by patient or spouse. Obtaining the sexual history requires tact and a sense of timing. The physician may elect to postpone detailed sexual history until later interviews, to restrict his initial inquiry to fairly general questions, or to wait until the patient provides an opening to this subject.

10. *Personality, Life Style, Interests*. The interviewer attempts to get a picture of the patient's general style of life, including his involvement with friends, clubs, and hobbies. If married, does spouse participate in patient's social life or do they tend to go their separate ways? Does patient feel lonely, excluded by others, or that he has difficulty in forming stable friendships? How does the patient imagine that his friends would describe him? Has the patient observed any recent change in his social activities and interests?

Does past history of patient's behavior suggest how well the patient tolerates stress or frustration? Has patient successfully pursued long-term goals? Has he tended to be sociable, seclusive, outgoing, secretive, realistically trusting, naive, suspicious, easily discouraged, tenacious, generous, stingy, disorganized, perfectionistic, steady, intellectual, excitable, emotional, impulsive, etc?

230

11. *Developmental History*.
   A. *Preschool Years*. To the patient's knowledge, was his mother's pregnancy with him and delivery of him free of complications? Quality and stability of family life during infancy and early childhood. How does the patient describe his parents, siblings, and his relationships with them during this and later periods of his life? Ages at which patient learned to walk and say sentences, if known. History of nightmares, eating problems, enuresis, encopresis, or any other serious behavior problem.
   B. *Early School Years*. Patient's recollection of his experiences and feelings when he began kindergarten and the first grade. Is there evidence of unusual separation anxiety? Is there a history of school phobia? Did he play much outside the home? Spend nights at friends' homes? Go to camp? Did patient have chums and did he develop hobbies during grade school years? How did he get along with classmates and teachers? What were his average grades? Did he have favorite subjects? Did he pass all grades and subjects in this and later periods of school? Is there a history of specific academic difficulties such as learning to read? Is there evidence of the patient's having been exceptionally active, restless, distractable?
   C. *Puberty and Adolescence*. Does patient recall first menstrual periods, acquisition of axillary and pubic hair, breast development, voice change, heightening of sexual feelings, early sexual interests in other boys or girls? If so, were these experiences relatively comfortable or pleasurable ones or were they associated with feelings of embarrassment, inadequacy, anxiety, or guilt? What is the person's experience with masturbation and associated attitudes and feelings? In obtaining the sexual developmental history, the physician exercises the same tact and precautions about timing as he does in obtaining the recent sexual history.
      History of dating behavior, crushes, important relationships with peers of both sexes, interest in intellectual pursuits, sports, part-time jobs. Was patient's adolescence relatively quiet or was it quite turbulent? Did he seem to make a successful shift of interests and emotional involvements to people and activities outside the home or did he remain dependent on his parents? Did he become involved in a continuing struggle with parents? Did he come into serious conflict with authorities?
   D. *Young Adulthood*. Did patient achieve a sense of knowing what he wanted to do in terms of work or further education? Did he make the transition from high school to college, or from school to work without major difficulty? Did he achieve a feeling of self-reliance, self-respect? Has the patient experienced a lasting love relationship with someone of the opposite sex? What are or were his

231

feelings and plans about marriage and parenthood during this period of his life?

PRESENT MENTAL STATUS

The mental status examination is carried out while one is interviewing the patient and is continued during the physical examination.

The psychobiologic processes illustrated in Figure 1 should be carefully evaluated in the course of the examination: (1) integrity of the sensory and motor apparatuses, (2) cognitive processes, (3) affective processes, and (4) functional concomitants of emotional states. This diagram represents a schematic attempt to depict human responses to internal and external stimuli as a psychobiologic system. This method of illustration carries the danger of oversimplification and of representing human behavior as a cut and dried, mechanical thing. While the schema does not explicitly depict psychologic defense mechanisms and unconscious motivation, it does not preclude these aspects of psychic functioning. Its purpose is to represent important functional categories which should be evaluated in examining the patient. The numerous two-way arrows in the figure signify the impressive way in which psychic processes influence each other.

These functions, illustrated in Figure 1, are evaluated by observing the patient's general appearance, the content and form of his speech, and nonverbal behavior. In conducting the mental status examination, the experienced physician will be guided by his own associations just as he is in any medical examination. For example, if the patient appears to have undergone recent weight loss the experienced physician will keep in mind the various features of severe depression (as well as other diagnostic possibilities) as he proceeds with the mental status examination. A grossly unkempt or disheveled appearance in a middle-aged, successful businessman immediately raises the possibility of recent personality change secondary to organic brain damage or severe depression with accompanying retardation and loss of interest. These and other hypotheses are tested as the examination proceeds.

OUTLINE OF MENTAL STATUS EXAMINATION

1. *Appearance, Speech, and Motor Behavior.* Various aspects of these three categories of data are included in some detail in the remainder of the mental status examination outline given below. Nevertheless, it is useful to record at the beginning one's general observations of the patient and any characteristics which more or less immediately strike the observer as being outstanding or important. This may include a

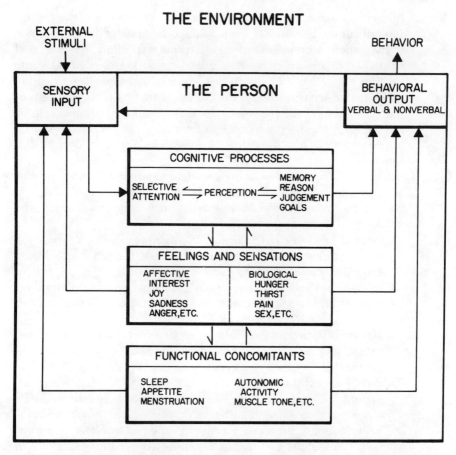

FIG. 1. The psychobiologic processes. (From Harvey AM, Johns RJ, Owens AH, Ross RS (eds): The Principles and Practice of Medicine, 19th ed. New York, Appleton, 1976)

description of (1) the patient's physical appearance, including height, weight, apparent age, state of health, grooming, attire; (2) demeanor or behavior suggestive of attitudes conveyed by terms such as friendly and cordial, cool but polite, taciturn, reserved, poised, seemingly ill-at-ease, avoids eye contact, rarely volunteers information, seems affected, looks worried, looks bewildered; (3) speech characteristics such as speed, vocabulary, inappropriate use of big words, ability to express feelings and thoughts, stammering, aphasia, echolalia, use of neologisms; and (4) motor behavior such as restlessness, hand-wringing, pacing, waxy flexibility, stereotyped activity, echopraxia, slowness, immobility, grimacing, tics, clumsiness, unusual gait (specify), tremor, choreiform movements, paralysis, and so on.

233

2. *Integrity of Sensory and Motor Apparatus*. Assessment of the organic integrity of the nervous system is an important part of the examination of the patient with emotional or behavioral difficulties. Evaluation of responses to spoken or written questions obviously must take into account the patient's ability to hear, to see, and to engage in appropriate motor behavior and speech. In the event that sensory deficits or motor weakness are present, do these conform to anatomic or physiologic patterns produced by organic lesions? Are there speech impairments, such as dysarthria or aphasia, indicative of organic dysfunction?

3. *Cognitive Processes*. The term cognition refers to all those psychic processes by which knowledge is obtained, retained, retrieved, and used. It therefore includes all aspects of perceiving, remembering, and thinking.

A. *General Level of Consciousness*. Is patient stuporous, sleepy, dull, or alert to his surroundings? Is he hyperalert, easily startled?

B. *Attention, Concentration, and Comprehension*. Does the patient listen to and understand questions? Is he easily distracted or preoccupied? Can he keep his mind on simple arithmetical tasks such as serially subtracting 7 from 100?

C. *Memory*. Is the patient able to recall events in the immediate, recent, and remote past? The immediate recall of a series of numbers tests concentration as well as memory.

D. *Perception*. This refers to a complex process by which one is meaningfully aware of objects, ie, their identity, location, size, and state of motion. Gross abnormalities of perception may take the form of hallucinations, illusions, misidentification of persons, abnormal body sensations, and apparent failure to perceive with one or another sensory modality.

E. *Orientation in Time, Place, Person, and Present Situation*. Correct orientation depends upon conscious awareness, perception, comprehension, and memory. It is well to remember that usually disorientation is only partial. For example, a patient may be accurately aware of the day of the week and month, but not the day of the month or the year; he may know what city he is in but not that he is in a hospital; he may know that he is in a hospital but not realize he is a patient. Therefore, when suspecting disorientation, the examiner carefully explores the various dimensions of personal identification, personal situation, place, time.

F. *Thinking and Speech*. In these categories are included all those remaining cognitive functions essential to successful adaptation to life: reasoning, ability to express oneself coherently, the accurate interpretation of reality, insight, judgment, and content of thought.

In expressing himself does the patient communicate the "goal idea" of his statement? Does he become lost in circumstantial details or does his line of thought become derailed by tangential associations? Does the patient talk rapidly and excessively? Does he appear to be experiencing a "flight of ideas"? Is his speech occasionally "blocked" so that he becomes suddenly silent and cannot remember what he was about to say?

To some degree, everyone's conception of reality is influenced by wishes, fears, other feelings, and mood. Is the patient's thinking so vulnerable to such influence that he has delusional concepts of the world around him, of himself, of the future? Is he suspicious of others? Does he feel persecuted, watched, controlled by outside influence? Is he grandiose or self-demeaning? Does he have delusions involving his body? What is his concept of the future?

Is the patient able to engage in abstract reasoning as manifested by his interpretation of proverbs? Can he solve simple arithmetic problems? Are his store of general information, grammar, and vocabulary in keeping with his educational background and station in life?

Does the patient have an understanding of his own condition and situation? In discussing recent activities and future plans does he appear to exercise sound judgment?

Is the patient preoccupied with particular topics? Does he have persistently recurrent ideas or obsessions? Is he compelled to engage in rituals to allay anxiety or to prevent harm to others? Does he recognize the absurdity of the compulsive rituals?

4. *Affective Processes.*
   A. *Display of Affect or Feelings.* Does the patient show feelings which are appropriate to the content of his speech? Does he appear to be "affectively flat"? Does he tend to be dramatic or histronic?
   B. *Anxiety.* Are there moments when the patient appears anxious, fearful, tense, or restless? If so, are there autonomic symptoms accompanying the anxiety states?
   C. *Mood.* This term refers to a prevailing and relatively enduring emotional state. There are many varieties and shades of mood. Among the important abnormal states of mood are depression and elation, which may be associated with a variety of behavioral manifestations.
   D. *Depersonalization and Derealization.* Does patient have the feeling that he or his body is unreal, that his surroundings are unreal? Does he feel estranged, suspended, or separated from his body or from his arms or legs, from his immediate environment, from his emotions?

5. *Functional Concomitants of Emotional States.*
   A. *Autonomic Concomitants of Anxiety.* Dilated pupils, tachycardia, pallor, sweaty palms, and tremor are not uncommon.

B. *Hyperventilation and Its Sequelae*. Paresthesias, giddiness, and tetany are common sequelae to hyperventilation.
C. *Eating Behavior*. Implied by evidence of weight loss or obesity and confirmed by history.
D. *Sleeping*. Does patient have difficulty in falling asleep? Does he awaken early? Does he sleep fitfully? Does he sleep more than is customary for him? Irresistible urge to sleep at inappropriate times?
E. *Miscellaneous*. Fatigue, diarrhea, constipation, sexual dysfunction, amenorrhea, urinary frequency, urinary retention, muscular tension, aching, and the like.

REFERENCES

1. Carr AC: Some instruments commonly used by clinical psychologists. In Freedman AM, Kaplan HT, Sadock BJ (eds): Comprehensive Textbook of Psychiatry, 2nd ed. Baltimore, Williams and Wilkins, 1975
2. Lisansky ET, Shochet BR: Comprehensive medical diagnosis for the internist. Med Clin North Am 51:1381, 1967
3. MacKinnon RA, Michels R: The Psychiatric Interview in Clinical Practice. Philadelphia, Saunders, 1971
4. Shafer R: Psychological tests in clinical psychiatry. In Redlich FC, Freedman DX (eds): The Theory and Practice of Psychiatry. New York, Basic Books, 1966
5. Sullivan HS: The Psychiatric Interview. New York, Norton, 1954
6. Whitehorn JC: Guide to interviewing and clinical personality study. Arch Neurol and Psychiatry 52:197, 1944

Chapter 17

Psychologic Aspects of Management

Management implies not only the application of specific therapeutic measures but also the design and implementation of a comprehensive, individualized program of care in the light of continuing evaluation of the patient.

GENERAL CONSIDERATIONS

Effective management of patients with psychiatric disorders rests upon the same basic principles that underlie the management of other medical disorders: (1) collection and analysis of data obtained from the history and observation of the patient, (2) delineation of specific problems, (3) the diagnosis of a specific clinical entity, (4) the discernment of those factors which have contributed to the development and continuance of the patient's illness, and (5) an assessment of the patient's assets and resources which may be key factors in the process of recovery.

The design and implementation of a comprehensive plan of care require all five of these steps. For example, in the management of a patient with depression it is essential to evaluate the "problem" of suicidal risk, for this will be an important determinant of planning treatment on an outpatient basis versus hospitalization. The patient's problems in functioning associated with psychomotor retardation will have an important bearing not only on one's psychotherapeutic approach, but also on the degree to which the patient is able to shoulder the demands of daily routine and work until symptomatic and functional improvement occur. The patient's attitude of trust in the physician, his confidence in the physician's ability, and an interested, cooperative spouse or family are invaluable assets in management.

Perhaps the most basic decision to be made by the physician is whether he will manage the psychiatric patient himself, with or without psychiatric consultation, or refer the patient to a psychiatrist.

PSYCHIATRIC REFERRAL

Which patients the primary physician refers to the psychiatrist and which patients he elects to manage himself depend in no small measure on the physician's schedule and on his interest and experience in the management of emotional disorders. Available time is a critical factor, especially when the therapeutic approach requires regularly scheduled visits of 20 to 30 minutes duration, once or twice a week, for several weeks or longer. Just as important, though less easily defined, is the issue of feeling interested, comfortable, and confident in the management of patients with psychiatric problems.

While there is, therefore, considerable variation among primary physicians regarding the indications for psychiatric referral, we believe that in general such referral is indicated when there is evidence of (1) psychosis or severe neurosis; (2) any serious behavioral problem, especially one which threatens the welfare of the patient or others; and (3) severe personality disorders, particularly when the patient himself expresses concern with his own attitudes and behavior. This obviously does not exhaust the possible occasions for psychiatric referral. There may be emotional disturbances primarily related to situational stress that warrant psychiatric referral or that warrant the services of a skilled social worker, marriage counselor, or a member of the clergy trained in pastoral counseling.

In referring the patient to a psychiatrist, whether for consultation or continued treatment, the physician must take care to (1) avoid giving the patient a feeling of being rejected, and (2) ensure that the patient understands the reasons for the referral and has had an opportunity to ask questions and express his views about it. The patient whose emotional disturbance is manifested by somatic symptoms and who has little awareness of significant emotional problems is apt to resist going to the psychiatrist if the referral is made prematurely; indeed, such a patient may feel that the physician has missed the diagnosis and he may seek help elsewhere. Thus, it is apparent that there are times when the physician may need to offer the patient several sessions, in which the results of the diagnostic evaluation are discussed and personal issues and feelings explored, in order for the patient to see the potential usefulness to him of psychiatric referral.

PSYCHOTHERAPY BY THE PRIMARY PHYSICIAN

Psychotherapy refers to a procedure in which the physician utilizes his relationship with the patient for the purpose of assisting him to recover from the emotional illness, to gain an understanding of his attitudes and problems in order to live a more satisfactory life, and to reduce the likelihood of future episodes of illness.[1,3,5,6] While the specific psychotherapeutic approach must be tailored to suit the individual patient and his particular problems, there are some principles and techniques of psychotherapy that are generally applicable and which will be presented here. The treatment aspects of specific clinical entities have been considered in the chapters devoted to them. Highly specialized treatment procedures, such as intensive, psychoanalytically oriented psychotherapy, and the details of specific behavior therapy techniques will not be described.

THE PHYSICIAN –PATIENT RELATIONSHIP

The most important element in psychotherapy is the establishment of a physician–patient relationship in which the patient feels that the physician respects him, listens to him, attempts to understand him, is truthful with him, and has a therapeutic intent. To emphasize the importance of these attributes of the therapeutic relationship may strike the reader as belaboring the obvious. But these elements of the relationship assume critical proportions for the patient who has low self-esteem; who feels bewildered, apprehensive, or discouraged; who is inclined to be distrustful of the motivations of others; or whose behavior and complaints have alienated him from others.

Transference   A substantial number of patients, whether they are receiving care for organic illness, emotional problems, or both, will sooner or later impute to the physician a set of attributes which he may not possess or which he may not possess to the degree imputed to him. Often this process, loosely referred to as transference, takes the form of idealization: the patient is convinced that his physician is the best diagnostician in the country, that his physician is an authority on everything, that he is a paragon of virtue and wisdom, that he must be a good husband, that his personal and family life is free of problems, that his memory is flawless (especially for anything the patient has told him), and that his devotion to the patient's health and welfare is boundless. There are endless variations on this theme and, needless to say, the less the patient actually knows about the physician the more readily does idealization develop.

There are usually several interrelated factors that contribute to the idealizing of the physician. An important one is that the patient's anxiety about his own illness and treatment is allayed, at least partially, if he perceives the physician as extraordinarily good and competent. Further, it is narcissistically gratifying for one's physician (or anyone or anything else that "belongs" to the patient) to be the best. And, finally, the human being tends to develop attitudes and feelings toward people in his current life similar to those he had toward persons in similar positions in his past; thus, the present feelings for the physician are in part displacements from those on whom he depended in the past such as parents, siblings, and other physicians.

The development of some degree of positive transference is probably essential to successful psychotherapy and this development ordinarily will occur if the physician displays reasonable dedication and competence. The physician is well advised to be mindful of the fact that in the presence of a strongly positive transference the patient may be highly susceptible to or influenced by the physician's verbal and nonverbal responses to the patient. In addition, the physician should expect that as the relationship goes on and as the patient has more experience with the physician, the transference image of the physician may be progressively replaced by a more realistic one.

Less commonly, the initial or early transference may be markedly negative in nature, the patient exhibiting any of a variety of attitudes such as questioning the doctor's competence or integrity, criticizing the physician, disregarding the therapeutic regimen, and so forth.

Sometimes the type of transference can be predicted by obtaining the history of the patient's past experiences with other physicians and other help-giving persons and authority figures.

The conducting of psychotherapy in the presence of a strongly negative transference can tax the ability and patience of highly skilled and experienced therapists. If the physician has reason to predict the development of a complicating negative transference he would be well advised to refer the patient to a psychiatrist. If a negative transference has developed, it is helpful for the physician to be aware of the transference nature of the patient's distorted view of him, ie, that the physician is the object of feelings that are unconsciously displaced from some other source. Such an awareness will help the physician to avoid becoming defensive, argumentative, or counterattacking, and to maintain a healthy degree of objectivity and distance. If, as is not uncommon, the patient expresses his negative feelings by an overdone reaction to some actual error or fault, the physician may matter-of-factly acknowledge the realistic basis of the patient's reaction and then follow with an equally matter-of-fact observation that the patient's feelings seem stronger than the present situation warrants. The physician can then ask the patient if the presently disturbing event seems at all familiar to him, ie, if he has had experiences like this before. Such an approach is often effective unless the patient's reality testing is momentarily swamped by the intensity of emotion such as rage. In the latter event, it is usually advisable to wait until the patient has cooled off a bit before attempting to enlist him in an objective review of his reaction.

The Therapeutic Alliance   There are many therapeutic situations in medicine in which the patient is in a relatively passive, receptive position, such as when treatment consists in the simple removal of a skin lesion. In conducting psychotherapy, however, such is not the case, for in the psychotherapeutic situation the patient and the physician are participants in a collaborative undertaking. In this collaborative endeavor the patient, his problems, feelings, conflicts, fantasies, and experiences are the continuing focus of interest.

An important intermediate or tactical goal of psychotherapy, therefore, is to establish a relationship in which the patient enters into a sort of partnership or alliance with the therapist. With the development of a therapeutic alliance, the patient strengthens his tendency and ability to observe himself, his own attitudes, feelings, and ways of behaving; and to notice connections between fluctuations in symptoms, emotions, and life

241

experiences. The patient himself may begin to discern problems which he had previously tended to dismiss or previously unnoticed modes of behavior which are largely maladaptive or self-defeating. He may become aware of problematic situations in his family which may or may not warrant the involvement of other family members in the therapy.

GOALS

The setting of one or more clearly defined goals is essential in order to develop a rational therapeutic approach. Flexibility, however, is required, for a goal at the outset of therapy may be modified or replaced by other goals as the work proceeds.

In general, the goals of psychiatric treatment fall into three groups: (1) relief of symptoms, (2) improved self-awareness, and (3) modification of behavior. While it is convenient for expository purposes thus to classify psychotherapeutic goals, it must be acknowledged that theoretically and in practice these three categories are not always sharply distinguishable. For example, many psychiatric symptoms can validly be regarded as types of behavior, such as the agitation or psychomotor retardation of depression. Further, the physician may aim for a goal which belongs in one category as a means of attaining goals which belong in the other categories, eg, improved understanding of one's own feelings, behavior, and problems may lead to more effective coping and thus to restoration of self-esteem and alleviation of other symptoms.

On the other hand, substantial symptom relief may occur in the course of therapy without any apparent change in the patient's awareness of his feelings or problems or in his ways of coping with problems. When this happens, the patient's improvement may have been related to factors other than treatment, or it may have been brought about by the supportive (including the transference) aspects of the physician–patient relationship. When the patient has achieved substantial relief from symptoms he may, of course, choose to terminate treatment regardless of whether any other therapeutic goals have been attained. When this occurs it is often wise simply to accept the patient's decision unless there are compelling reasons to do otherwise.

PSYCHOTHERAPEUTIC PROCEDURES

The Setting and Contract   The setting refers to the environment in which the psychotherapy sessions are conducted. Privacy is of basic importance. One cannot expect the patient freely to discuss his feelings and personal problems if the office door is ajar or if he is aware that conversation is audible in the adjoining room even with the door shut. Sound-proofed rooms are uncommon in many modern buildings, but lack of soundproofing can often be overcome by use of low-volume music or a background of "white sound" in the adjoining room.

Some attention to the seating arrangement during the therapy session is warranted. In general, it is helpful for both parties to be seated in comfortable chairs with no intervening structure, such as a desk, between them. Most patients and therapists are more comfortable if the chairs are not directly facing each other but are set at right or oblique angles. Some patients prefer to sit close to the therapist and others are more comfortable at a distance.

The therapeutic contract refers to an agreement or understanding of the terms of treatment which should be made explicit at the beginning of therapy. This includes such matters as the schedule of visits, fees, anticipated vacations, and so forth.

There is often an advantage to establishing a regular schedule of visits. To arrange return visits on an "as needed" basis may set up a situation in which symptom recurrence (or persistence) is inadvertently rewarded. Regularly scheduled visits, on the other hand, take place independently of symptomatic status. The frequency and duration of interviews are determined by the clinical situation and the realities of the physician's schedule. Weekly sessions are often useful, particularly at the beginning of treatment, in order to allow continuity of therapy to develop. Acutely disturbed patients initially may need to be seen more frequently than once a week. Much may be accomplished in relatively brief interviews of, for instance, 20 to 30 minutes' duration.[2] With regard to duration of treatment, the physician may find it useful to suggest a tentative limit, such as 10 to 12 weekly sessions. This may need to be reevaluated as the end of the time period approaches. There are apt to be occasions when relatively brief psychotherapy has revealed indications for referral of the patient for more extended and intensive treatment.

When the physician has set up a schedule of appointments, he, as well as the patient, is expected to abide by it. To keep a patient, who has a regular weekly appointment, waiting for an hour is to invite resentment, for it is a way of saying that the physician's time is important but the patient's is not. If a delay occurs and was unavoidable the physician should inform the patient of that fact.

Many psychotherapists find it useful to present to the patient the concept that the scheduled visit is a block of time that the physician has reserved for the patient. Therefore, should the patient arrive 10 minutes late for a 30-minute session, only 20 minutes of the session would remain available. Similarly, some understanding should be reached about the desirability of the patient and physician giving each other advance notification when a visit is to be canceled.

The Interview   In a general sense, the guiding principles of interviewing during a series of psychotherapy sessions are the same as those described in Chapter 16. However, the actual content, focus, and style of the interview vary considerably, depending upon the patient's needs and interests at any particular point in time and the personality of the therapist.

For example, at the beginning of treatment of a severely depressed patient, the physician strives to be supportive, and to avoid long interviews or excessive probing or questioning which may aggravate the patient's already painful feelings of guilt or inadequacy. In this circumstance the physician may choose simply to ask the patient to describe how he is feeling and to report any change in his condition; he may wish to change the dose of the antidepressant drug and to so inform the patient; he may invite the patient to bring up any concerns which come to mind without implying that the patient must think of some; he may choose to offer the patient some encouraging comment, being careful to avoid false reassurance; and so forth. Later in the course of treatment, as the depression improves, the patient may or may not indicate that he has this or that "problem" in his life, perhaps connected with the depression, which he wishes to discuss with the physician.

On the other hand, a different approach is required in the management of the patient who manifests emotional problems by means of somatic symptoms and hypochondriacal worries. The primary physician is often in a better position to engage such patients in psychotherapy than is the psychiatrist, because he is in a position to deal authoritatively with the patient's concerns about his physical health. In the course of managing the patient whose defenses predominantly consist of somatic symptoms or worries, the physician may from time to time deem it helpful to repeat a relevant part of the physical examination or laboratory test. If at such times the physician feels that the examination or test will be "negative" he should share that prediction, and, later, the results of the examination or test, with the patient. Such an approach should be supplemented by an effort to ascertain the psychologic issues that are related to the somatic symptoms. But how does the physician get past the somatic defenses and into the underlying emotional problems?

A useful technique, the application of which has been extensively described by Shochet and Lisansky, is that which Deutsch labeled "the associative anamnesis."[4] The physician begins the interview by encouraging the patient to talk about those issues or concerns which are uppermost in his mind. The patient will often begin with a description or recitation of somatic symptoms. In that event, the interviewer accepts the implicit fact that the patient's anxiety is momentarily leading him to focus on physical symptoms or problems. The interviewer listens, however, for spontaneous references (associations) that the patient may make to emotions and/or life circumstances while he is describing his symptoms, eg, the day of the week, the place, or the person he was with when he noticed a particular symptom such as headache, backache, dizziness, or tenseness. At an opportune moment, the interviewer expresses an interest in hearing more about the particular circumstance which the patient had thus spontaneously associated with his symptom.

As therapy progresses and as the relationship deepens, the physician's display of interest in associated feelings and problems becomes important to the patient, and reinforces his tendency to delve into the important issues of his life which are related to his illness. Occasionally, the patient's associations may lead him toward a topic which arouses anxiety. He is then apt to shift the conversation to another topic. In most instances, it is advisable simply to take note of but not comment upon this defensive avoidance, unless it is felt that the patient is ready to hear such an observation and to make constructive use of it.

Specific Techniques   SUGGESTION   The power of suggestion usually increases as the physician–patient relationship solidifies, particularly if a positive transference develops. Some patients are much more easily influenced by suggestion than are others. The physician should use suggestion sincerely, sparingly, and with a degree of subtlety commensurate with the sophistication of the patient. The physician may use suggestion unconsciously as when he prescribes, with an air of confidence, a particular medicine. He may use suggestion quite deliberately (though with due regard for the patient's sensitivity) in managing a patient with acute conversion symptoms.

CONDITIONAL REINFORCEMENT OF BEHAVIOR   Although the theory and techniques of operant conditioning will not be described, it is apparent that in conducting psychotherapy the physician will find it useful to reinforce useful and healthy behavior (verbal and nonverbal) in ways which are suitable for the individual patient. For example, the physician may reinforce the hypochondriacal patient's mention of nonsomatic concern by a show of appreciative interest; this may be simply a change of facial expression, leaning forward a little, or a verbal response. At times, reinforcement may be done somewhat more obviously as when the patient reports a constructive change he has made in his life. It is also possible of course to reinforce undesirable behavior. An example was given above when it was pointed out that scheduling the patient on an "as needed" basis may have the effect of rewarding the development of symptoms.

REFLECTION OF FEELINGS   It is sometimes very supportive for the therapist to let the patient know that he has observed how the patient feels, ie, to "reflect" the patient's feelings back to him. This may be done simply by saying that the patient looks depressed or sad or tense or angry, or by commenting that the experiences or situations which the patient has just described must have been rather upsetting or must have made the patient feel such and so. Frequently the accurate reflection of the patient's feelings has the effect of momentarily loosening defenses, allowing a transient surge of affect to be expressed; this may contribute to the patient's feeling of being understood by the physician and of being in rapport with him.

VENTILATION OF FEELINGS (ABREACTION)   Abreaction refers to a process in which the patient experiences an outpouring of pent-up feelings while relating emotionally charged experiences in the recent or remote past. While abreaction may give the patient only a temporary feeling of relief from tension, it may also be educational in that it gives him increased awareness of how certain experiences can remain emotionally charged and have a continuing influence on one's sense of well-being.

CLARIFICATION   The physician asks the patient to express more clearly or completely his feelings and thoughts about a particular issue, or encourages the patient to clarify the relationship between certain events in his life. If the physician has discerned the repetition of certain kinds of behavior in certain situations, he may point this out to the patient, thus helping him to develop a clearer grasp of his own behavioral history. The physician may point out that a given somatic symptom developed about the time a certain event occurred in the patient's life. Clarification, when done persistently and with due regard for proper timing and for the patient's sensitivity, can facilitate the therapeutic alliance in which the patient himself becomes a self-observing partner. Care must be taken, however, to avoid overly zealous clarification which would deprive the patient of the opportunity to clarify his feelings and problems for himself.

DESENSITIZATION   Desensitization refers to a process in which the patient becomes less sensitive to or fearful of a topic, object, or situation by means of gradually increased exposure to it. Psychotherapy which respects the patient's defenses and which starts with feelings and thoughts that are most accessible ("on the surface" of the patient's mind) can be thought of as carrying out a process of desensitization along a broad front. Desensitization, however, usually refers to a more narrowly focused, rigorously systematic method of treatment of specific phobias.

MANIPULATION   Manipulation refers to a procedure in which the therapist takes advantage of emotions, wishes, or values existing in the patient in order to promote the therapeutic process. For example, in dealing with a patient who prides himself in being independent and who is probably discomfited at the notion of needing help, the physician may quietly emphasize the point that in psychotherapy the patient does a great deal of the work, perhaps even most of it. Manipulation, as we have defined it here, is doubtlessly used much more extensively in interpersonal transactions than most of us realize. The dependent patient, the patient who craves the therapist's approval and who fears rejection by him, may be easily influenced by the therapist. This influence (manipulation), which capitalizes on the patient's needs and fears, must always be used strictly in the patient's best interest, such as for the promotion of self-understanding, the modification of self-defeating behavior, or relief from suffering. The concept of manipulation has gained an unsavory reputation because it is often used only to refer to those occasions when the manipulator uses it for his own purposes with no regard for the welfare of the other person.

ALTERATION OF ENVIRONMENT   In treating the emotionally ill patient, it is always important to carefully assess his current total life situation, particularly his relationships with the immediate family, the relationships between other members of the family as these are perceived by the patient, and the patient's situation at school or work. Tensions and conflicts within the family may have contributed significantly to the patient's illness and be strong factors working against his recovery. When this is the case, members of the family or the entire family may be in need of counseling or therapy. Situational stresses related to family problems and occupational or economic difficulties may require the service of a skilled social worker who is not only trained in counseling techniques but who is also thoroughly familiar with social agencies and valuable resources in the community. Many members of the clergy are trained in pastoral counseling and they, like the family physician, are often in an excellent strategic position to be of help to distressed individuals and families.

REFERENCES

1. Balint M: The Doctor, His Patient and the Illness. New York, International Univ Press, 1957
2. Castelnuevo-Tedesco P: The Twenty-Minute Hour. Boston, Little, Brown, 1965
3. Levine M: Psychotherapy in Medical Practice. New York, Macmillan, 1942
4. Shochet BR, Lisansky ET: New dimensions in family practice. Psychosomatics 10:88, 1969
5. Strupp H: On the technology of psychotherapy. Arch Gen Psychiatry 26:270, 1972
6. Whitehorn JC: Understanding psychotherapy. Am J Psychiatry 112:328, 1955

Chapter
18

Psychopharmacologic Aspects
of Management

Antimanic Agents
  Dosage and Administration of Lithium Carbonate
  Lithium Toxicity
Insomnia: Brief Comment on Management
  Assessment of Sleeping Disturbances
  Some Common Sleep Disturbances of Adults
  Management

Modern psychopharmacologic agents are specific and potent aids in the management of patients with psychiatric problems. These medications are widely used, and the physician may encounter them in two ways: (1) he may choose a psychotropic medication as part of his own management of a patient; and (2) he may learn, while treating a patient for another condition, that the patient has been taking a psychotropic medication. In either instance the physician will need to know the therapeutic effects of the medication, its side effects, and its possible interactions with other drugs.

There are many psychotropic medications, but they fall into a limited number of major classes: antianxiety drugs, antipsychotic drugs, antidepressant drugs, antimanic drugs, and sleep-producing drugs. Within each of these classes, the therapeutic effects of the various medications are similar, although medications of a particular class may differ substantially in type and severity of side effects. In instituting chemotherapy the physician first decides which class of medication is indicated and then which specific drug in that class he chooses to prescribe.[2,3,5]

Thus, the decision to use psychotropic medications requires several steps.

1. An accurate diagnostic assessment must be made.
2. Goals of management, such as the alleviation of anxiety, depression, or the psychotic manifestations of schizophrenic illness, must be set.
3. The physician then decides if a psychotropic medication will help to achieve the desired goal.
4. If he so decides, he then chooses the specific medication and explains his prescription to the patient.
5. On return visits he judges the effects of the medication and adjusts the dosage accordingly.

We shall discuss only a few representative drugs in each class. Thorough knowledge of these few medications can provide a sound base for clinical practice, and a reference for comparison with data about other drugs. Dose ranges given are those generally recommended for adults. Older patients (above age 60) usually require less medication than younger patients; it is prudent to begin the treatment of the older patient with smaller doses and to increase the dosage gradually.

ANTIANXIETY DRUGS

Among the drugs available for the treatment of anxiety, the benzodiazepines, chlordiazepoxide (Librium) and diazepam (Valium), are currently the most widely prescribed. They are generally safer than and at least as efficacious as other readily available antianxiety drugs such as meprobamate (Miltown, Equanil) and hydroxyzine (Vistaril, Atarax).

INDICATIONS

Not all patients with symptoms of anxiety require medication. In Chapter 12, anxiety neurosis, in its acute and chronic forms, was described. It should be noted that anxiety symptoms do not always connote neurosis, for everyone experiences transient anxiety or tension in stressful settings such as facing examinations, deadlines, confrontations with superiors, and the like. The presence of mild to moderate anxiety in such situations can be viewed as a normal part of arousal and adaptation to environmental challenge. If, however, anxiety is severe and prolonged, it interferes with normal functioning and the patient seeks and needs relief.

As was emphasized in Chapter 12, psychotherapeutic intervention alone is often effective in treating patients with anxiety, and has the advantage that when the patient has learned to identify and cope with feelings and problems connected with the anxiety he has reduced the likelihood of future recurrence of symptoms. Further, anxiety symptoms often come and go "spontaneously" and, therefore, symptom alleviation following drug administration may sometimes be a matter of coincidence. Such a coincidence, however, is apt to be viewed as a therapeutic effect by the patient and thus lead him to think that he needs the drug more than he really does.

Nonetheless, patients in whom anxiety is severe, persistent, and interferes with performance, especially those who have not responded to initial psychotherapeutic sessions, often need medication as an adjunct to psychotherapy.

The benzodiazepines, especially chlordiazepoxide and diazepam, are also widely used in the treatment of alcohol withdrawal syndromes (see Chap. 9).

When used in small doses, the antianxiety drugs are quite safe. Early in treatment, especially when higher doses are employed, sedative effects are regularly encountered. For this reason, and because of wide variation among individual responses to these drugs, it is wise to apprise the patient of these side effects which are especially apt to occur in the first few days of treatment. If the patient drives a car or engages in other hazardous activity he should be warned of possible drowsiness during the day.

The other two major problems which can be encountered in the use of antianxiety drugs are drug dependence and the effects of deliberate overdose by the suicidal patient.

Psychologic dependence on any drug can occur and this is particularly true of a drug which alleviates discomfort such as anxiety or tension. However, there are significant differences among the antianxiety drugs with regard to the development of tolerance and physical dependence. Of the antianxiety agents listed in Table 1, physical dependence is most apt to develop with meprobamate when used in doses exceeding the recommended amount for long periods of time. The withdrawal syndrome occurs more quickly and is more apt to be severe when meprobamate is abruptly discontinued than is the case with the other agents. Further, like the barbiturates, meprobamate induces the development of drug-metabolizing enzymes to a greater extent than is the case with ben-

Table 1. Approximate Total Daily Dosages for Antianxiety Drugs

BENZODIAZEPINES

Chlordiazepoxide (Librium)	15–100	mg
Diazepam (Valium)	6–40	mg
Oxazepam (Serax)	30–120	mg
Clorazepate (Tranxene)	7.5–60	mg

ANTIHISTAMINES

Hydroxyzine (Atarax, Vistaril)	30–200	mg

PROPANEDIOLS

Meprobamate (Equanil, Miltown)	1200–1600	mg

zodiazepines, and therefore tolerance on a metabolic basis is more apt to occur.

The relative lack of tolerance and the long plasma half-life of some 24 to 48 hours of the benzodiazepines (as compared to a plasma half-life of 10 hours for meprobamate), probably contribute to the lesser likelihood of physical dependence on the benzodiazepines and the fact that withdrawal symptoms are slower to appear and are comparatively less severe following discontinuance of these drugs. However, as noted in Chapter 10, a withdrawal syndrome, including organic psychosis and seizures, has been reported following abrupt discontinuance of benzodiazepines when taken in high daily doses.

Of great practical importance is the fact that it is very difficult to commit suicide with overdoses of the benzodiazepines alone, whereas meprobamate has been fatal when taken in doses as small as 20 g.

The antianxiety drugs are not indicated in the treatment of patients with severe or endogenous depression, and indeed may aggravate depressive symptoms. With the exception of delirium tremens (and possibly other states associated with withdrawal from general CNS depressants), the antianxiety drugs are not used in the treatment of psychoses, other drugs (the antipsychotic and antimanic drugs) being the agents of choice for these conditions.

DRUG INTERACTIONS

CNS depressant drugs tend to have a potentiating effect on each other when used concomitantly. For example, the depressant action of alcohol or a major tranquilizer such as a phenothiazine may be enhanced if the patient is also taking an antianxiety agent.

DRUG CHOICE, DOSAGE, AND ADMINISTRATION

There is probably not a great deal of difference between the anxiety-reducing effects of meprobamate and those of the benzodiazepines. However, the benzodiazepines are preferred over meprobamate because they are safer. Further, the benzodiazepines are probably more effective than either phenobarbital or hydroxyzine, when these drugs are given in doses that do not induce excessive drowsiness. As Hollister[2] has pointed out, however, the patient's preference based on previous experience is a factor to be taken into account in choosing an antianxiety drug. The physician is hesitant to change a patient from a drug which the patient has used responsibly and has found to be acceptable and beneficial, even though the drug may not be the physician's first choice.[2]

The usual dose ranges of these drugs when used for alleviation of anxiety are shown in Table 1. It is advisable to use the least amount of drug that is found to be effective. With that in mind, the drug is started at a low dose and gradually increased to the lowest amount necessary to achieve a reasonable degree of symptomatic relief. Although the benzodiazepines have long plasma half-lives, their peak actions are usually two to four hours after an oral dose. Therefore, it is often useful to administer the daily amount of these drugs in three or four divided doses through the day, or during that part of the day when the patient is most apt to experience discomfort. The dosage schedule for diazepam (Valium) may range from 2 to 10 mg, one to four times a day; and for chlordiazepoxide (Librium), 5 to 25 mg, one to four times a day. Valium may be preferred over Librium in patients who have symptoms suggestive of heightened muscle tension because of its muscle-relaxing effect.

The physician keeps in mind the fact that it is not feasible to strive for complete relief of anxiety symptoms through chemotherapy alone. Substantial though incomplete symptom relief may promote confidence in the physician and promote the development of a therapeutic relationship between patient and doctor, in the context of which the patient can be fruitfully encouraged to develop greater understanding and ability to cope with problems related to his anxiety.

To reduce the likelihood of psychologic and physical dependence it is desirable to administer the drug in time-limited courses. However, this may be easier said than done when the patient's anxiety state persists or continually recurs over a long period of time. Discontinuance of the drug should be gradual, especially when high doses have been employed or administration has continued for longer than a month.

ANTIPSYCHOTIC DRUGS

There has been an extraordinary proliferation of antipsychotic drugs since the introduction of chlorpromazine in the mid-1950s. Among the older, well-established members of this group are the phenothiazines, the butyrophenones, and the thioxanthenes. More recent additions include dihydroindolones and dibenzoxazepines. All of these agents are effective in the treatment of the psychotic manifestations of schizophrenic illness, and all can produce extrapyramidal symptoms if given in sufficient dosage. There are considerable differences among these drugs in potency (dosage) and some differences among them in type and severity of side effects such as sedation and hypotension.

INDICATIONS

These drugs have sometimes been referred to as "major tranquilizers." However, that is a misnomer, for these agents do not produce tranquility in either normal or psychotic subjects. These powerful drugs, which are sometimes associated with serious side effects, are not recommended for use as hypnotics or in the management of neurotic anxiety. They are reserved for major psychiatric disorders as follows: (1) schizophrenic illness; (2) mania (as an adjunct to lithium carbonate); (3) depression in which there is agitation, severe anxiety, or psychosis; (4) severe panic states, especially when associated with psychosis; and (5) organic brain syndromes in which there are serious behavioral disturbances and/or psychotic manifestations.

These drugs are not the agents of choice in the treatment of syndromes secondary to withdrawal from CNS depressants. In the management of panic or psychosis caused by ingestion of hallucinogenic substances, it is prudent to avoid the use of phenothiazines because of possible interactions affecting cardiovascular function. In this circumstance, if a drug is deemed necessary, haloperidol or a benzodiazepine may be used (see Chaps. 7, 9, and 10).

SIDE EFFECTS AND ADVERSE REACTIONS

Sedation   These drugs vary considerably in the degree to which they produce sedation. Among the phenothiazines the tendency to produce sedation is inversely correlated with the antipsychotic potency of the drug. Thus, the high-dose, low-potency phenothiazines such as chlorpromazine (Thorazine) are more sedating than are the low-dose phenothiazines such as perphenazine (Trilafon), trifluoperazine (Stelazine), and fluphenazine (Prolixin). Similarly, the relatively low-dose nonphenothiazine agents such as haloperidol (Haldol), molindone (Moban), and thiothixene (Navane) have weak sedative effects. Loxapine (Loxitane) and chlorprothixene (Taractan) are intermediate in sedating action.

Postural Hypotension   The antipsychotic agents have alpha-adrenergic blocking action as manifested by their tendency to produce postural or orthostatic hypotension. This is an important side effect, especially when dealing with elderly patients or those who have a history of cardiovascular disorder. It is of practical interest that among the antipsychotic drugs the tendency to produce postural hypotension parallels the tendency to produce sedation as described in the preceding paragraph.

Neurologic Effects   Extrapyramidal side effects are the most common problem with antipsychotic medications. They should be detected and treated quickly, since subtle extrapyramidal effects may make patients discontinue their antipsychotic medications.[6] Most can be managed with either a reduction in drug dosage or an antiparkinsonian medication. Rigidity, akathisia (stiffening and restlessness, especially in legs), and dystonia (torticollis, oculogyric crisis) may occur early in treatment, or after a sudden increase in antipsychotic dose. If relief is urgently needed, intramuscular diphenhydramine 50 mg, or benztropine mesylate 2 mg, will give quick results. The patient can then be placed on benztropine mesylate (Cogentin) 2 mg by mouth once or twice daily.

Parkinsonism, with rigidity, tremor, and slowing of movements, also may result from use of the antipsychotic medications. Again, an antiparkinsonian medication will be effective in counteracting this problem. Some advocate beginning all patients on such a medication when they begin antipsychotic medications. Since not all patients on antipsychotic medications will develop extrapyramidal side effects, this is a preventive measure that is questionable. Furthermore, the additive effects of antipsychotic and antiparkinsonian medications can make patients most uncomfortable with dry mouth, blurred vision, and even the possibility of central atropinic toxicity. Thus, we do not recommend routine use of antiparkinsonian medications in treatment of schizophrenia. Even after a patient is placed on these medications to treat specific side effects he should be checked periodically, since the extrapyramidal effects often lessen after several months of treatment, and the extra medication may no longer be necessary.

Tardive dyskinesia gets its name from the observation that it tends to occur after a relatively long period of treatment and is manifested by repetitive movements of the mouth and tongue (grimacing, smacking, chewing, tongue protrusion) and sometimes of the trunk, extremities, and feet. Elderly women may be particularly susceptible to this condition. The syndrome may first appear when the drug is being lowered or discontinued. It may slowly disappear weeks or months after chemotherapy has been stopped. Recurrence of the psychosis for which the drug was originally given may, of course, militate against discontinuing the drug. Since the incidence of this condition may be related to the total amount of drug received over a period of time, it seems prudent to administer these drugs at the lowest effective dosage and for no longer than necessary. However, if the psychotic disorder for which the drug is prescribed is severe and unremitting, the physician may have no feasible alternative to continuing chemotherapy. In treating chronically ill patients some psychiatrists periodically schedule drug-free days ("drug holidays") in an effort to reduce total drug consumption, but the efficacy of this in preventing tardive dyskinesia has not been proven.

Anticholinergic Effects   Anticholinergic effects include dry mouth, tachycardia, constipation, and blurred vision. Often these symptoms are mild and may remit after a few weeks of continuing drug usage. In predisposed individuals, urinary retention may occur. Inhibition of ejaculation sometimes develops and is particularly associated with the use of thioridazine. The anticholinergic action of these drugs may also cause exacerbation of untreated glaucoma. In delirium or toxic psychosis secondary to another anticholinergic agent (such as a tricyclic antidepressant), antipsychotic drugs should not be used; instead, the causative agent should be removed.

Metabolic and Endocrine Effects   Gynecomastia, diminution of libido, and weight gain may occur.

Miscellaneous Complications   Cholestatic jaundice is now very rare. Agranulocytosis, to which elderly, white women seem most susceptible, occurs infrequently and usually within the first two or three months of treatment. Skin eruption and photosensitivity may be associated with these drugs.

There are rare instances of sudden death in patients receiving a phenothiazine, suggesting the possibility that the major tranquilizers may have the potential of precipitating ventricular fibrillation. Disturbances in myocardial repolarization are sometimes associated with thioridazine administration, and therefore it may be prudent not to administer thioridazine with a tricyclic antidepressant.

Pigmentary retinopathy may occur when thioridazine is given in doses exceeding 800 mg per day.

DRUG CHOICE AND DOSAGE

If the patient has a past history of good therapeutic response to a specific drug, the same drug should be selected if the present illness is similar to that for which the patient was previously treated. Other factors to be considered in choosing a drug are

1. Desirability or undesirability of sedating action in the management of the patient
2. Avoidance of hypotensive side effect in elderly patients and patients with cardiovascular disease
3. Physician's familiarity with a particular drug.

If allergic or idiosyncratic responses occur with the use of an antipsychotic agent, another drug belonging to a different chemical category may be used; thus an allergic response to a phenothiazine, for example, would lead the physician to select a nonphenothiazine such as haloperidol.

Drug dosage must be individually determined. The comparative therapeutic potency of various antipsychotic agents is given in Table 2. When possible, especially when managing elderly patients, it is advisable to begin with a low dose and increase this gradually to attain the desired symptomatic response. Sometimes, however, this approach is not feasible.

In managing an acutely disturbed schizophrenic patient one may choose a sedating drug, such as chlorpromazine, especially if excitement and sleep deficit are part of the clinical picture. In such a case, a starting oral dose of 400 to 600 mg of chlorpromazine per day may be employed. The physician may also choose to initiate treatment of the acutely disturbed patient with the intramuscular administration of 25 to 50 mg of chlorpromazine, in which case the patient's blood pressure should be monitored for two hours following the injection. If the patient does not respond adequately to the initial daily dose, it can be increased by 30 to 50 percent the following day. As the patient improves, the dose may continue to be increased once or twice a week until it is felt that optimal response has occurred. For most hospitalized patients the maximum dosage of chlorpromazine is 1800 mg daily. Going beyond this amount generally will not give better results; a patient who has not responded to 1800 mg of chlorpromazine daily for two weeks should be switched to another

Table 2. Comparative Therapeutic Potency of Antipsychotic Medications

GENERIC NAME	TRADE NAME	DOSE IN MG EQUIVALENT TO 100 MG CHLORPROMAZINE
Chlorpromazine	Thorazine	100
Thioridazine	Mellaril	100
Triflupromazine	Vesprin	30
Acetophenazine	Tindal	24
Perphenazine	Trilafon	8
Trifluoperazine	Stelazine	2.5
Thiothixene	Navane	4.4
Haloperidol	Haldol	1.6
Molindone	Moban	6
Loxapine	Loxitane	10
Fluphenazine HCl	Prolixin/Permitil	2

medication, either another phenothiazine or a nonphenothiazine such as haloperidol.

After the patient's psychotic symptoms are significantly alleviated, the dosage of chlorpromazine can often be reduced, over a period of three or four weeks, to a level of 300 to 600 mg per day. At this stage of treatment many patients will be better on a less sedating medication, such as perphenazine, 24 to 48 mg per day. These medications can be given once daily, usually at bedtime.

After several weeks at these intermediate dose levels, the medication can be reduced further to the lowest effective level, ie, the maintenance dose. This is often in the range of 8 to 32 mg of perphenazine, given in a single dose in the evening. A single evening dose is relatively easy for the patient to remember and disrupts daily routine less than do several divided doses per day.

Deciding whether to continue the patient with schizophrenic illness on a phenothiazine indefinitely or to stop after six to 12 months is based on several factors. After a first schizophrenic episode medication can usually be discontinued after the patient has been relatively symptom-free and able to perform usual activities for several months. On the other hand, the patient who has had several psychotic episodes or one who does not respond to early symptoms of relapse by returning for treatment is a candidate for indefinitely prolonged antipsychotic maintenance medication. In these cases, the physician weighs the disadvantage of recurrent psychotic episodes against possible undesirable effects of prolonged medication such as tardive dyskinesia.

Those patients who do not take oral medication reliably can benefit from the long-acting phenothiazine, fluphenazine decanoate (Prolixin decanoate), which may be administered intramuscularly at two- to four-week intervals, usually at a dose of 25 mg.

DRUG INTERACTIONS

Drug interactions include the incompatibility of phenothiazines with guanethidine, and the additive effect when more than one drug with anticholinergic action are given concurrently. Since guanethidine and phenothiazines act on the same nervous system receptors, they cancel each other's effects by competition.

The central atropinic syndrome may result from additive effects of any number of medications with atropinic effects; these include antipsychotic agents, antidepressants, and antiparkinson drugs. Presenting symptoms of the atropinic syndrome are fever, excitement, visual hallucinations, along with peripheral signs of atropinism such as pupillary dilation, dry mouth, and dry skin. Therapy with physostigmine 1 to 4 mg by intramuscular or intravenous route is rapidly effective.[5] Since the syndrome can mimic a psychotic relapse in a schizophrenic patient, for which therapy would be quite different, one should consider this diagnosis with patients taking large doses of two or three medications in the above classes.

As already mentioned in the discussion of antianxiety drugs, the CNS depressant actions of the antipsychotic agents and other depressants such as hypnotics, alcohol, and minor tranquilizers are potentiated when they are used concomitantly.

ANTIDEPRESSANT DRUGS

There are two types of antidepressant drugs available: tricyclic compounds and monoamine oxidase (MAO) inhibitors. In this country, MAO inhibitors are rarely used in treating depression, except in those instances where the patient has failed to respond to treatment with the tricyclic antidepressants. This policy has been adopted because there appears to be no particular therapeutic advantage to the MAO inhibitors, and the risk of serious adverse reactions is somewhat greater than with the tricyclics.

There are several tricyclic antidepressant drugs available. Since there are no clearly demonstrated differences in their effectiveness in alleviating depression, the practitioner does well to become familiar with two or three established drugs. The drugs we have chosen to consider are imipramine (Tofranil) and amitriptyline (Elavil). These drugs are thought to exert their therapeutic action by blocking the reuptake of serotonin or norepinephrine or both in CNS synaptic clefts. However, it has not been proved that this action accounts for the effect of these drugs on depression.

INDICATIONS

In Chapter 14, the clinical characteristics, classification, and general principles of management of depressive syndromes were discussed. It was noted that the antidepressant medications seem to be particularly effective in depression in which there are "endogenous" features, namely, psychomotor retardation, loss of energy, anhedonia, diurnal variation in mood, and vegetative signs such as constipation, loss of appetite, and insomnia with early morning awakening. Importantly, endogenous depressions are "autonomous" in the sense that they are disproportionate in severity and duration to the precipitating circumstance and do not respond significantly to environmental changes or psychologic intervention.

SIDE EFFECTS

The tricyclic antidepressants have anticholinergic effects. Dry mouth and constipation commonly occur. Urinary retention may also occur and these drugs should be used cautiously or not at all in individuals predisposed by urinary tract pathology to this complication. These drugs are contraindicated in patients with narrow angle glaucoma.

Cardiac arrhythmia and postural hypotension are not uncommon; hence these drugs should be used cautiously in elderly patients and patients with a history of a cardiovascular disorder.

Rarely, the atropinelike action of the tricyclics is associated with the development of a toxic psychosis or delirium. This serious complication requires immediate cessation of the drug and usually requires hospitalization. The administration of physostigmine (which crosses the blood-brain barrier) is rapidly effective in ameliorating this condition.

DRUG INTERACTIONS

As with the antipsychotic drugs, the tricyclic antidepressants inhibit the antihypertensive action of guanethidine by competing for the same receptor sites. The anticholinergic action of these drugs is additive when they are used in conjunction with other anticholinergic drugs. It has been suggested that thioridazine not be used with the tricyclics because of the possibility of increased incidence of cardiac arrhythmia.

DRUG CHOICE, DOSAGE, AND ADMINISTRATION

Imipramine and amitriptyline have similar actions, similar dose schedules, and a similar time-course of therapeutic effect. Both require one to three weeks to produce a significant alleviation of depressive mood, although improvement in appetite, increased interest in activities, and more restful sleep commonly occur earlier. The other available tricyclic antidepressants do not act more rapidly than imipramine and amitriptyline.

Amitriptyline is somewhat more sedating than imipramine and therefore may be the preferred agent for the depressed patient who has severe insomnia. Considerable tolerance to the sedating action of the tricyclic drugs develops after a few days of continued usage. An occasional patient may exhibit unusual susceptibility to the sedating action of the tricyclic drug. For such a patient it may be helpful not only to give the entire dose in the evening but to maintain dosage at a relatively low level until tolerance has developed.

In the young or middle-aged patient, the usual starting dose is 75 mg in the evening, increasing the dose by daily increments of 25 mg to a level of 150 mg per day. It is important to inform the patient of the drug's sedating action and of the likelihood that there will be a delay of one to three weeks before he notices substantial improvement in the depression. The patient must be told of the importance of taking the medicine regularly. If after about ten days, the patient has no change in sleeping pattern, appetite, or general level of energy, the dose should be increased by 50 mg per day up to an effective level, but not above 300 mg per day. It may be noted that a common error made in using these drugs is that of failure to prescribe them in doses that are high enough to be effective.

These drugs should be used more cautiously with elderly patients. The initial evening dose for the elderly patient may be 10 to 25 mg, with maintenance at this level until it is observed that the patient is tolerating the drug without adverse side effects. Then a gradual build-up to 75 to 100 mg per day can usually be achieved; it may be wise to give the drug to elderly patients in divided daily doses rather than in a single bedtime dose in order to lessen the likelihood of postural hypotension upon arising in the morning.

Following remission of the depression, drug treatment should be continued for several months, but the exact length of time required is not known. If there is an earlier history of depression with spontaneous remission one may be guided by that and administer the drug for a comparable period of time. In the absence of such a history, it seems reasonable to begin dosage reduction about three months following remission. If maintenance at a reduced level (such as 50 percent of the original effective therapeutic dose) for a month or two does not result in symptom return, further reductions can be instituted gradually until discontinuance is achieved. An occasional patient requires maintenance at a low dosage level (25 to 50 mg per day) indefinitely.

Failure to respond to a particular drug after six weeks of treatment at adequate doses indicates a need to modify the therapeutic regimen. In such an event it is advisable for the physician to refer the patient to a psychiatrist for continued management. The psychiatrist in turn has several options available to him, such as switching to another drug and/or hospitalization.

ANTIMANIC AGENTS

Lithium ion, provided in the form of lithium carbonate, is effective in the management of the acute manic phase of manic-depressive illness, and in reducing the frequency and severity of future psychotic relapses which are characteristic of that illness. Management of acute mania and long-term prophylactic management of the patient with manic-depressive illness are generally carried out by psychiatrists experienced in the use of lithium carbonate. The acutely manic patient almost always requires psychiatric hospitalization and often an antipsychotic agent, usually one of the phenothiazines, is used in the initial phase of management until therapeutically effective blood levels of lithium are obtained.

The general physician needs to be aware of the way in which lithium carbonate is administered to manic patients and its pharmacologic properties for (1) he may be asked to provide medical clearance prior to the institution of lithium carbonate, (2) he may be asked to assist the psychiatrist in the management of the patient with lithium toxicity, and (3) he may encounter a patient who is receiving lithium carbonate who consults him regarding incidental medical problems.

Prior to beginning lithium administration, the physician will do a general medical examination. Lithium is excreted virtually entirely by the kidneys and its rate of excretion is affected by water and salt intake and excretion. Therefore, it is important to determine that renal function is adequate. Patients with cardiovascular conditions that require low-salt diets and diuretics are not good candidates for lithium carbonate treatment, since the risk of lithium toxicity in such patients is considerable. Any condition that results in dehydration and/or sodium depletion such as fever, vomiting, and diarrhea, may increase the blood lithium concentration to toxic levels. Therefore, when such conditions occur the lithium carbonate should be temporarily reduced or discontinued, depending upon the severity of the intervening illness. At such times, the lithium blood level should be carefully monitored. Since the chronic administration of lithium carbonate is sometimes associated with thyroid enlargement or changed thyroid function and elevated WBC count, it is prudent to obtain a baseline determination of thyroid status and the WBC count.[1,5]

DOSAGE AND ADMINISTRATION OF LITHIUM CARBONATE

The management of the patient with acute mania requires psychiatric hospitalization. The psychiatrist usually employs a phenothiazine in the initial phase of treatment in order to obtain rapid, though usually partial, control of manic behavior. While this is being done, medical examinations are conducted to rule out any medical contraindications to the use of lithium carbonate.

In the management of acute manic episodes, the patient should attain a blood level of 1.0 to 1.5 mEq of lithium per liter. The dosage required to reach this blood lithium concentration varies considerably among individuals, but generally initial daily doses of 1200 to 1800 mg of lithium carbonate, administered orally in three or four divided doses, are sufficient. During this initial phase of management blood levels are obtained three to five times weekly, blood being drawn in the morning 12 hours after the last dose.

With remission of the acute manic episode, the daily dosage of lithium carbonate is reduced in order to attain a maintenance level in the range of 0.7 to 1.2 mEq/liter. For most patients, this requires a daily oral dosage of 600 to 1200 mg per day in three or four divided doses. When the lithium blood level has been stabilized it should be routinely checked every two or three months. As already noted, in addition to regular monitoring of the patient's mental state and blood lithium level, the physician must be alert to any intercurrent condition that affects fluid and electrolyte balance. Any disorder that includes impairment of renal function, vomiting, diarrhea, prolonged elevations of body temperature, profuse sweating, or reduction of fluid intake calls for discontinuance of lithium until the condition is corrected.

LITHIUM TOXICITY

Mild symptoms of toxicity may occur at blood levels that are within the therapeutic range. They are more apt to occur at levels above 1.5 mEq/liter and become progressively more severe as the blood level increases.

Early signs of toxicity include anorexia, nausea, polyuria, thirst, and a fine tremor of the hands. Patients should be instructed to call their physician if these occur. With increasing lithium intoxication the following signs and symptoms develop: vomiting, diarrhea, muscle weakness, muscle hyperirritability (fasciculations, twitching, sometimes clonic movements of limbs), somnolence, slurred speech, seizures, confusion, stupor, and coma.

The management of mild lithium toxicity may simply require temporary discontinuance of lithium and monitoring of blood lithium levels. In cases of more severe toxicity hospitalization may be indicated; serum electrolytes and an EKG should be obtained and vital signs carefully monitored. The intravenous administration of fluids and electrolytes is required in severe toxicity, especially when nausea and vomiting are present. Forced diuresis to enhance lithium excretion with the use of urea or mannitol may be considered. In critically ill patients peritoneal dialysis or hemodialysis may be required.

INSOMNIA: BRIEF COMMENT ON MANAGEMENT

The use of medication is but one approach in the management of insomnia. It is important to note that hypnotic drugs tend to be overprescribed in the management of patients with insomnia. Like any other symptom, insomnia requires thoughtful diagnostic assessment and, when possible, a plan of treatment directed at its underlying causes. When the latter approach is used, hypnotic drugs may not be necessary at all or will only be used as a limited and small part of the management plan.[4]

ASSESSMENT OF SLEEPING DISTURBANCES

An accurate description of the patient's sleeping pattern should be obtained, including difficulties (or lack of them) in falling asleep or remaining asleep through the night and any recent change in time of awakening in the morning. A careful review of the patient's physical health, drug history, emotional state, and life experiences concurrent with onset, remissions, and exacerbation of the insomnia should be obtained.

SOME COMMON SLEEP DISTURBANCES OF ADULTS

Among the common contributory causes of difficulty in falling asleep at night are (1) the excessive use of caffeine-containing beverages, (2) taking naps in the afternoon or after dinner (which the patient often justifies on the basis of lack of nighttime sleep), (3) emotional tension, and (4) physical discomfort. The latter two etiologic factors may also be associated with disturbing dreams and frequent awakening during the night. Less common conditions associated with difficulty in getting to sleep and staying asleep are hyperthyroidism, withdrawal from CNS depressant drugs, and the use of stimulating drugs such as cocaine and amphetamines. Insomnia is often among the early signs of moderate to severe depression, and frequently takes the form of early morning awakening with or without difficulty in falling asleep and fitful sleeping.

In assessing sleep function, it is well to keep in mind that with advancing age people tend to awaken more frequently during the night and to take brief naps during the day.

MANAGEMENT

The basic aims of treatment are directed at those factors which may be contributing to the insomnia such as the alleviation of any physical condition which may be contributing to sleep-interfering discomfort, eg, dyspnea or pain. The patient should be encouraged to limit ingestion of caffeinated drinks and confine their usage to the first half of the day. Daytime or evening naps should be discontinued by the nonelderly patient who complains of insomnia. Regular physical exercises during the early part of the day are often helpful in inducing a pleasant degree of tiredness at day's end, especially for individuals with sedentary occupations. In tense or worried individuals, counseling or psychotherapy may be needed in order to resolve underlying problems. In addition, many tense persons benefit from being taught how to achieve muscular relaxation, by alternately tightening and relaxing muscle groups beginning with the toes and working up to the facial musculature. In insomnia associated with depression, it is the latter on which therapeutic efforts are focused.

Hypnotic drugs are of very limited use in the treatment of insomnia. Most of them lose their effectiveness after a few days unless progressively larger doses are used. Further, most hypnotic drugs suppress REM sleep, and this in turn may contribute substantially to feelings of tension and restlessness. Therefore, if the patient is already taking hypnotic medications, it is advisable that the dose be tapered to zero over a period of several days. (In the event of daily dosage sufficient to cause addiction, considerable caution is indicated. See Chapter 10.) The patient whose hypnotic drug is being discontinued should be advised that although he may not sleep perfectly the first night or so, his sleep pattern will most likely return within a few nights.

If it is deemed necessary to use a hypnotic drug for a brief period while other therapeutic measures are being taken, flurazepam (Dalmane) is reasonably effective and is one of the safer agents available both in terms of addictive potential and hazards of overdose. The average nighttime dose of flurazepam is 30 mg, although 15 mg often suffices for the elderly patient.

REFERENCES

1. American Psychiatric Association: The current status of lithium therapy. Report of the APA task force. Am J Psychiatry 132:997, 1975
2. Hollister LE: Clinical Use of Psychotherapeutic Drugs. Springfield, Ill, Thomas, 1973
3. Klein DE, Davis JM: Diagnosis and Drug Treatment of Psychiatric Disorders. Baltimore, Williams and Wilkins, 1969
4. Regenstein QR: Treating insomnia. A practical guide for managing chronic sleeplessness, circa 1975. Compr Psychiatry 17:517, 1976
5. Shader RI (ed): Manual of Psychiatric Therapeutics. Boston, Little, Brown, 1975
6. Van Putten T: Why do schizophrenic patients refuse to take their drugs? Arch Gen Psychiatry 31:67, 1974

PART
V

PSYCHOSOMATIC MEDICINE

Chapter
19

Introduction to Psychosomatic
Concepts

Definition
Psychosomatic Medicine: A Controversial Field
A Brief Historical Perspective
Clinical Categories Included in Psychosomatic Medicine

DEFINITION

The term "psychosomatic" has been used in several ways. Alexander[1] suggested that it be used to designate a method of approach to research and therapy, in which techniques and concepts appropriate to somatic processes are coordinated with those appropriate to psychologic processes. For example, a psychosomatic investigation of gastric function might include (1) "somatic" techniques such as those involved in observing gastric motility, determinations of the acidity and enzyme content of gastric secretions, and observations of the influence of sympathetic and parasympathetic stimulation on gastric function; and (2) psychologic techniques such as noting the effect of certain kinds of environmental stimuli or subjective emotional states on gastric function.[1]

The term psychosomatic has also been used to describe any physiologic process or disease in which it has been demonstrated or postulated that psychologic factors play an important, though not exclusive, causative role. One or two decades ago, it was not uncommon for the term to be used in this restricted sense and, if one wished to refer to a mental or emotional state caused by somatic factors, it was logical to reverse the term and use the adjective "somatopsychic." The latter term, however, has not gained wide usage.

At this time, psychosomatic medicine has gained a rather broad connotation and refers to the study and treatment of those conditions which are related to the interaction of psychic and somatic phenomena. Later in this chapter we will enumerate the various categories of clinical phenomena included in psychosomatic medicine, thus defined.

It may be noted that the term psychosomatic has been criticized because, some contend, it has become so inclusive as to be almost useless. Among the laity, particularly, psychosomatic is often used synonymously with psychologic or psychiatric. The view has also been expressed that psychosomatic implies mind–body dualism, ie, that there is an entity, the "psyche," which is separate and distinct from the "soma." This particular criticism is ironic when one considers that virtually all serious students of psychosomatic medicine have gone to some pains to point out that they regard psychologic functions, such as perception, feeling, and thinking, to be as much a part of body (somatic) physiology as are circulation of the blood and respiration. It is of great practical value, however, to distinguish psychic processes from other physiologic processes because they lend themselves to study by psychologic methods. At this stage of our knowledge it is not feasible, for example, to discern what a man is thinking by physiologic monitoring of his cerebral cortex, but one may gain an approximate notion of his thought content by talking with him and observing his behavior.

PSYCHOSOMATIC MEDICINE: A CONTROVERSIAL FIELD

Not only has the term psychosomatic been in dispute but the field of psychosomatic medicine itself has often been rife with controversy. There are a number of reasons for this. Perhaps a very basic one relates to an almost universal tendency to regard psychologic difficulty not only as a mark of failure or inadequacy, but also as something for which the individual is responsible or is "to blame" and which he could rectify if only he would. If that is our attitude toward the individual with emotional problems, it might well seem cruelly unjust to regard an obviously organic illness as psychosomatic, for that would seem to contradict our wise and humane tradition of not blaming a person for being ill and of not holding him responsible for his own cure except for the responsibility of seeking expert medical help. In actuality, of course, the psychosomatic concept of disease does not diminish our humane concern for the patient, but indeed gives it added dimension. Nevertheless, some laypersons and physicians seem to feel that to regard a given disorder as psychosomatic is to regard it as less real and less respectable than an organic illness in which psychologic factors are not etiologically implicated. This deep emotional resistance doubtlessly promotes the often-observed, exaggerated skepticism of psychosomatic hypotheses, even when they are supported by carefully controlled observations.

On the other side of the coin, however, much of the controversy about psychosomatic medicine has stemmed from valid criticisms of unwarranted research claims, exaggerated therapeutic expectations, ludicrous misapplications of psychoanalytic concepts to organic processes, and from the fact that often there are serious methodologic problems in the scientific validation of psychosomatic hypotheses. Some of these difficulties were more prominent two or more decades ago than at present and will be further discussed in the following section.

A BRIEF HISTORICAL PERSPECTIVE

The influence of spirits, gods, and sin upon bodily health was widely accepted in antiquity and in certain later epochs and cultures. Not infrequently, the roles of priest and healer were combined in ancient times and remain so in some isolated contemporary cultures and subcultures. Job's friends insisted that his bodily afflictions, as well as his other misfortunes, were punishments for his sins. The ancient Greeks attributed the phenomena of various diseases, as well as practically everything else, to the gods. Hippocrates not only espoused a nonmystic and rational (in the terms of his day) approach to the theory and practice of medicine, but he seems to have had a point of view which, to a degree, was consistent with modern psychosomatic concepts. He believed that brain lesions could cause mental illness, that humoral changes in the body influenced emotional states, and that, sometimes, emotions could somehow bring about physiologic or bodily changes.

In the eighteenth century, following the decline in belief in witchcraft and demoniac possession, there was another return to a nonmystic, rational approach to the understanding and treatment of mental illness. This newly revived approach not only included a strong emphasis on humane treatment of the mentally ill, as exemplified by Pinel and Tuke, but also took account of the role of physical and psychologic factors in the development and treatment of mental illness. Further, the possible role of psychologic factors in physical health was also seriously considered. Georg Ernst Stahl, at the beginning of the eighteenth century, did not concur with the prevailing tendency to dichotomize the human being into body and mind, pointed out that passions and affects had significant effects on the body, and expressed his belief that emotions could interfere with recovery from physical disease. Later, Lieutaud (1703–1780) commented that the mind and body influence each other and added that the extent of that influence was not known.[6]

In the nineteenth century, a nonmystic, scientific approach to mental disorders continued to prevail but, with the impact of impressive advances in cellular pathology and bacteriology, there appears to have been a tendency to turn away from serious consideration of the role of psychologic variables in the pathogenesis of disease states. It is probable that adherence to the scientific method tended to be equated with the study of tangible, physical variables which could be observed by examination of the living patient, or at autopsy by gross anatomic inspection and chemical, bacteriologic, and microscopic examination of tissues and tissue fluids. There seems little doubt that the hard won victory of the scientific method over the not-so-distant medieval mysticism and superstition was to be carefully guarded against any reintrusion, whether real or apparent, of anything that suggested a postulated role of psyche, spirit, or soul in the causation of medical diseases. This organicism also became evident in attitudes toward mental or emotional disorders, which were assumed to be like any physical disease. Not surprisingly, this point of view, which held sway well into the twentieth century, resulted in a high degree of compatibility, perhaps even a fusion, between psychiatry and the rest of medicine.

In the early decades of the present century, a swing toward the psychosomatic approach in medicine developed, mainly under the influence of Freud's psychoanalytic theories and, to a lesser extent, the psychobiology of Adolf Meyer.

The revival of psychosomatic medicine in this century has thus far been a biphasic one, in the sense that by the 1950s it had probably reached a zenith of popularity among the laity and physicians, followed by a period of disappointment and skepticism which is now being replaced by a less dramatic, but more solid, scientific development of the field. Undoubtedly a substantial part of the rapidly developing enthusiasm for psychosomatic medicine in the second quarter of this century was an outgrowth of the enormous influence which the relatively young field of psychoanalysis gained in psychiatry and among the intellectual avant garde of that period; it seemed that psychoanalytic methods of interpretation contained an explanatory power with extraordinarily wide applicability not only to the neuroses and psychoses, but also, though with apparently greater limitations, to an increasingly long list of psychosomatic disorders. The psychoanalytic ability to understand illnesses of all sorts seemed to carry with it commensurate heuristic promise and therapeutic optimism. There were restraining voices, for example, that of Whitehorn, who emphasized the difference between understanding the "meaning" of illness and understanding its cause.[5]

Meyer's psychobiology, with its emphasis on understanding the whole person, his biologic equipment, the interplay between biologic givens and life experiences in the development of reaction patterns, and the environmental setting in which maladaptive reaction patterns or illness occurred, became particularly influential in the Unitied States and England in the first half of this century. It helped to develop a fertile field in which a psychobiologic or psychosomatic approach to medical illnesses, as well as psychiatric ones, could flourish.

Another impetus came from the experience in both world wars in which not only psychiatrists but also other medical specialists were impressed with the large numbers of young men who were not able to serve in the armed forces because of psychiatric disability or who became emotionally ill while on active duty, some under the stress of combat conditions and others in less severely stressful circumstances. Somatic manifestations of emotional stress, including apparent effects on organic disorders, such as the effect of air raids on the frequency of malarial attacks in a previously exposed population, made an impression on military physicians which did not vanish when they returned to civilian life.

As already noted, the early and mid-twentieth century enthusiasm for psychosomatic medicine was followed by a period of rather widespread disenchantment. This occurred for a variety of reasons, including the following:

1. *The inappropriate application of psychoanalytic interpretation.* Symptoms and signs, which were manifestations of altered physiology or tissue damage, were sometimes interpreted as having primary symbolic meaning, ie, in these instances it was explicitly or implicitly postulated that the alleged symbolic content was of primary, etiologic significance. Thus, fever (a hot body) might be interpreted as representing sexual excitement; a swollen, infected finger symbolized a tumescent penis, and so on. Such ludicrous misuse of psychoanalytic theories may well have struck many physicians as a return of medieval mysticism in secular guise. Franz Alexander, whose work will be discussed further, was one of the pioneers in psychosomatic medicine who helped to differentiate between those somatic symptoms which do have symbolic meaning from the outset and those which do not. The latter type may become endowed with symbolic significance *secondarily*, as in the case of a man who came to feel that the absence of a leg, as a result of surgical amputation, "meant" that he had been deprived of manliness or virility. In such an instance, preexisting insecurity about his status as a man undoubtedly was crucial in the patient's so interpreting his loss, but equally clearly was unrelated to the gangrene which necessitated the amputation.
2. *Psychosomatic medicine was inadvertently oversold.* The new insights into human behavior which psychoanalysis offered seemed to promise a new, powerful therapeutic approach not only to traditional psychiat-

273

ric illnesses, but also to those disorders which were considered to be psychosomatic. While psychotherapy has its rightful place in the management of psychosomatic illness, it is not a cure-all. The elucidation of psychologic factors in the genesis of peptic ulcer, for example, did not lead to a curative psychologic approach, applicable to all patients with peptic ulcer. The leading scientific investigators never made the claim that it would, but nevertheless a high expectation of definitive therapy developed among many people who were, of course, disappointed.

3. *Methodologic problems in psychosomatic research.* In view of the great breadth of the field included in psychosomatic medicine, it is to be expected that the aims and methods of psychosomatic research are quite varied. A large group of investigations, both in clinical settings and in the laboratory, have attempted to demonstrate a correlation between psychologic variables, on the one hand, and the incidence, time of onset, pathogenesis, and recovery from medical illnesses, on the other. Other investigations, which, to be sure, are related to these, have focused primarily on the emotional or behavioral reactions to medical illness and its associated variables, such as hospitalization and other aspects of diagnostic evaluation and treatment. An intriguing but difficult line of investigation addresses itself to the mechanisms by which psychologic processes influence (and are influenced by) other physiologic processes, ie, how to make the "leap from the mind to the body," as Freud put it.[2-4]

There are numerous and serious methodologic problems in all of these areas of investigation, but we will confine our discussion to several which are encountered in the area of research first mentioned, that in which the investigator attempts to discern the influence of psychologic variables on the development and course of physical illnesses. The problems encountered include the following.

1. In studying a patient with a given disorder, it may be difficult to distinguish between those psychologic characteristics which are primary and those which develop as a reaction to the illness. One approach to this problem is that of observing the patient prior to the illness.

2. In all scientific investigations it is necessary to exclude observer bias. Ideally, this is best accomplished by separating psychologic assessment (independent variable) from assessment of physiologic changes or illness (dependent variable). Although there are notable examples in which this has been done, it is a technique which poses grave problems if the psychologic variable under scrutiny does not lend itself to an operational definition which allows a high degree of validity and reliability of observations. For example, it is no simple matter to develop a valid, reliable, operational definition of "stress" or "significant object-loss."

3. Theoretically, one can test a psychosomatic hypothesis, eg, that psychologic factors contribute to the cause of a disease, by removing or altering the psychologic variable through treatment, such as psychotherapy. Among the problems with this approach is that, frequently, once an organic disease process is initiated it is possible that other factors quickly enter the picture and influence or perpetuate the disorder.

4. Animal experimentation has been useful in psychosomatic research as it has been elsewhere in medicine. Nonetheless, it is often risky to apply the results of animal experiments to human beings, particularly when one is dealing with psychologic, emotional, or symbolic phenomena which are associated with higher cerebral function and which, in some respects, may well be uniquely human.

Having enumerated some of the methodologic difficulties encountered in psychosomatic research it is noteworthy that none of these problems is insurmountable, as is evidenced by the number and variety of excellent investigations conducted in the last 25 years.

CLINICAL CATEGORIES INCLUDED IN PSYCHOSOMATIC MEDICINE

As noted earlier in this chapter, psychosomatic medicine, in its broadest sense, refers to the study and treatment of those conditions which are related to the interaction of psychic and somatic phenomena. As thus defined, psychosomatic medicine includes the following.

1. *Psychologic reactions to physical illness.* This includes the whole range of emotional and behavioral responses to physical illness and those circumstances or experiences associated with illness, such as what the illness means to the patient, patient behavior which facilitates or impedes treatment and recovery, the psychologic impact of the environment in which treatment occurs, and the relationship between the patient and staff (Chaps. 3 to 6).

2. *Disturbances resulting from disorders affecting brain function.* In this category are included not only the acute and chronic brain syndromes, but also those disorders in which the effect on cerebral function may result in psychologic disturbance with or without symptoms of mental confusion (Chap. 11).

3. *Medical complications of maladaptive behavior.* This group includes the numerous physical complications associated with various behavior patterns: alcoholism, drug dependence, overeating, self-starving as in anorexia nervosa, suicide attempts, accident proneness, antisocial behavior, and so on (Chaps. 7, 9, 10, and 12).

4. *Emotional disorders manifested by somatic symptoms with no organic basis.* This includes not only conversion hysteria and hypochondriasis, but also emotional illness such as depression in which somatic symptoms may be the presenting or even the predominant complaint (Chaps. 13 and 14).

5. *Physiologic concomitants of emotional states.* This group includes the manifestations of autonomic activity associated with emotional states, such as acute anxiety or fear, and physiologic concomitants not dependent upon autonomic innervation, such as increased muscle tone associated with emotional tension. As a convention, these conditions, in which there is alteration of function without structural change or tissue damage, will be referred to as functional disorders.

6. *Psychosomatic diseases.* In this book, we choose to use the term psychosomatic disease to refer to an organic disorder in which there is structural change or tissue damage, and in which it is postulated that psychologic factors contribute importantly to etiology.

It may be noted that the conditions included in the last two categories, namely, functional disorders and psychosomatic diseases, are usually collectively referred to as psychophysiologic disorders. These are discussed in Chapter 20.

REFERENCES

1. Alexander F: Psychosomatic Medicine. Its Principles and Applications. New York, Norton, 1950
2. Lipowski ZJ: Review of consultation psychiatry and psychosomatic medicine. III. Theoretical issues. Psychosom Med 30:395, 1968
3. Mendelson M, Hirsch S, Webber CS: A critical examination of some recent theoretical models in psychosomatic medicine. Psychosom Med 18:363, 1956
4. Meyer E: The psychosomatic concept, use and abuse. J Chronic Dis 9:298, 1959
5. Whitehorn JC: The concepts of "meaning" and "cause" in psychodynamics. Am J Psychiatry 104:289, 1947
6. Zilboorg G: A History of Medical Psychology. New York, Norton, 1941

Chapter
20

Psychophysiologic Disorders

A classic illustration of the interrelationship between psychologic, neurophysiologic, and peripheral physiologic processes is afforded by a study of the organism's response when confronted by a serious threat.

Cannon and Bard demonstrated the occurrence of "sham rage" in the decerebrate animal and the crucial role of the hypothalamus in the generation of the rage reaction.[2] Subsequent studies have implicated the hypothalamus, and cortical and subcortical structures known collectively as the limbic system, in emotional arousal.[9] Through the connections between the hypothalamus and the autonomic nervous system, the arousal of anger or fear characteristically is accompanied by sympathetic discharge with widespread effects throughout the body, preparing the organism for action such as fight or flight.

Hypothalamic discharge mediated through the autonomic nervous system is also involved in other physiologic responses appropriate to a variety of essential behaviors such as eating, sexual activity, and relaxing. In addition, because of neural and humoral relationships of the hypothalamus with the pituitary, nerve impulses arising in association with emotional arousal can have relatively long lasting physiologic effects virtually anywhere in the body; these nerve impulses also ascend to the cerebral centers involving conscious awareness and motor activity.

From the psychologic viewpoint, a critically important observation is that there is often enormous variability among human subjects in the way they interpret and respond to virtually identical situations or stimuli. A situation which may be extremely stressful or threatening for one person may be less so for a second subject and not at all for a third. The way in which a person responds to a given stimulus is a function of his current mental set and the sum of all his past experiences. Because of man's ability to abstract and thus to endow objects with symbolic meaning, the responses of human beings to environmental stimuli are far more variable than are those of laboratory animals.

Further, civilized man, unlike animals "in nature," is often threatened or provoked in situations where neither running nor fighting serves his purpose, even though his emotional and physiologic reactions prepare him for just such behavior. Even the verbal discharge of emotion may not be in the person's best interest under certain circumstances. It is possible that the prevalence of psychophysiologic disorders in modern man is related to the fact that evolution equipped him with certain basic physiologic responses to stress that facilitated behavioral responses (such as fight or flight), which were adaptive at various primitive stages of his evolutionary development but which would be highly maladaptive in present society.

As noted in Chapter 19, there is a group of disorders which appear to be physiologic concomitants of emotional states or to be triggered by emotional factors, and in which the resulting alteration of function is not accompanied by significant structural change or tissue damage. We have chosen to refer to these psychophysiologic conditions as "functional disorders."

On the other hand, we have chosen to refer to those psychophysiologic conditions in which there is significant structural change or tissue damage as "psychosomatic diseases," and to consider them separately from the functional disorders. This is a matter of semantic convention for expository convenience. The psychosomatic diseases, as we have thus defined them, have generally sparked much more controversy than have the functional disorders.

FUNCTIONAL DISORDERS

In Table 1, the more common functional disorders are grouped according to the physiologic system which is primarily involved. Many of these functional syndromes occur quite frequently and therefore it is not unusual for a patient to have, or to have a history of, two or more functional disorders involving the same or different systems of the body.

It is apparent that many of the disorders listed in Table 1 involve functions which are strongly influenced by the autonomic nervous system, such as sweating, heart rate and rhythm, vasoconstriction and vasodilation (migraine), intestinal motility, and so forth. However, some functional disorders do not appear to be primarily related to autonomic dysfunction. Such is the case in the hyperventilation syndrome which results in respiratory alkalosis and its physiologic consequences. Similarly, sustained contraction of skeletal muscle, which may accompany emotional tension, gives rise to pain in the involved part of the body, such as occipitonuchal or temporal headaches, and backache.

DIAGNOSIS

The diagnosis of a functional disorder is made by (1) the presence of symptoms and signs characteristic of a particular functional syndrome, (2) the exclusion of organic disease through appropriate physical examination and laboratory procedures, and (3) the presence of chronic tension, episodes of anxiety, and/or stressful life situations.

Caution must be exercised in judging the diagnostic significance of a correlation between anxiety or stress on the one hand and the occurrence or exacerbation of symptoms on the other. While the presence of such a correlation does support the diagnosis of functional disorder it by no means proves it, since symptoms arising from organic lesions also may be influenced by the emotional state of the patient.

Of considerable practical aid in diagnosis is the fact that most functional

279

Table 1.   Functional Disorders Associated with Psychologic Stress

PHYSIOLOGIC SYSTEM	SYNDROME
1. Cardiovascular	Migraine headache
	Vasovagal syndrome (fainting)
	Tachycardia, palpitations
2. Gastrointestinal	Irritable colon
	The following symptoms may occur singly or together: anorexia, nausea, vomiting, abdominal cramps, diarrhea, constipation, aerophagia
3. Genitourinary	Menstrual disturbances
	Difficulties in micturition; frequency (in both sexes), hesitancy (in males)
	Dyspareunia
	Anorgasmia
	Impotence
	Delayed ejaculation; premature ejaculation
4. Muscular	Pain secondary to increased muscle tension: occipital or bitemporal headaches, backaches, myalgia in various muscle groups
	Fatigue
	Tremor
5. Respiratory	Hyperventilation syndrome
	Bronchospasm
	Dyspnea
6. Skin	Urticaria
	Hyperhidrosis
	Pruritis

(From Harvey AM, Johns RJ, Owens AH, Ross RS (eds): The Principles and Practice of Medicine, 19th ed. New York, Appleton, 1976.)

disorders tend to be either chronic or intermittently present over a period of time, usually without evidence of significant progression in severity of the condition. In contrast, many organic disorders of relevance in differential diagnosis are either of self-limited duration or, if chronic, tend to show evidence of progression over a sufficient period of time. There are of course exceptions to this generalization. An example in which this generalization does apply would be the long-term course of functional headaches, such as tension headache or migraine, when compared with headaches secondary to brain tumor or untreated hypertension.

The management of functional disorders includes (1) measures taken to alleviate specific symptoms and (2) measures directed at the psychologic factors underlying the disorder.

In those disorders in which relatively severe discomfort is a feature of the functional disorder, careful attention to symptom relief is of paramount importance and generally precedes or accompanies that part of the therapeutic regimen which is aimed at influencing associated emotional factors. It would be obviously inappropriate, for example, to attempt to treat a patient with severe migraine by means of psychotherapy alone. Failure to attend effectively to the alleviation and prevention of the migraine attacks by adequate medication would likely cause the patient to lose confidence in the physician and to seek help elsewhere. The more severe the discomfort or the incapacity associated with the particular functional disorder the more important is the issue of attempting to afford the patient at least partial symptomatic relief, even though the underlying psychologic factors may not be affected by symptomatic treatment. It is possible, of course, that effective symptom relief will result in the patient's not having much interest in exploring those aspects of his feelings and experiences which are connected with the functional disorder. Quite commonly, symptomatic therapy alone is only partially effective and this fact, in combination with an awareness of anxiety, depression, or other disturbing feelings or problems, may render the patient accessible to an approach aimed at the psychologic roots of his difficulty.

Psychotherapy in treatment of the functional disorders is often helpful in several ways. Occasionally, the symptom history itself reveals an obvious clue to the area of the patient's life which merits especially careful exploration; this is the case when symptoms are exacerbated regularly in certain types of family, social, or occupational situations. A correlation of that type may lead to useful exploration which reveals that the setting in which symptoms recur is typically associated with certain kinds of feelings such as feeling thwarted or frustrated, angry, helpless, uncertain, sad, or anxious. Verbal expression or "ventilation" of feelings is sometimes associated with symptom relief, eg, the verbal expression of hitherto suppressed (or repressed) anger with the patient identifying what the anger is all about may result in rapid abatement of tension headache. More important in the long run, however, is the delineation of important, relevant personal issues about which the patient is in some way emotionally stressed, and the development of more satisfying and effective ways of coping with these issues. Thus, the successful psychotherapeutic approach to the management of functional disorders may not only help to relieve and prevent symptoms of the disorder, but may also facilitate the patient in achieving a less tension-ridden, more satisfying life.

Since anxiety is so commonly present in patients with functional disorders, a minor tranquilizer is commonly used. Chlordiazepoxide is sometimes helpful; diazepam may be preferred in those cases in which muscle tension is an important factor. Care should be taken to avoid physical dependence and to minimize psychologic dependence on the drug. With that in mind, it is helpful to prescribe the minor tranquilizer in the lowest daily dose that is effective and to prescribe the drug for limited "courses," such as three or four weeks rather than indefinitely. It is also helpful to explain to the patient that he may expect the tranquilizer to reduce tension and tension-related discomfort but not completely to eradicate it.

In severe functional disorders or those which do not respond to treatment, psychiatric consultation is advisable.

PSYCHOSOMATIC DISEASES

BASIC CONCEPTS AND THEORIES

As previously noted, psychosomatic disease refers to those disorders in which there is structural tissue damage and in which it is postulated that psychologic factors importantly contribute to etiology. A variety of theories and investigative approaches have emerged in recent decades, only several of which will be reviewed in this brief discussion.

Most psychosomatic theories have the following postulates in common:

1. Multicausality of disease. Most organic diseases are the result of a number of factors, some related to the organism and others to the environment. In psychosomatic diseases, psychologic factors are held to be important or necessary, but not sufficient, in the causation of disease.
2. Certain psychologic reactions to life events are associated with physiologic changes that promote development of disease. Most theories stress the point that premorbid personality development is an essential consideration because, as noted earlier, an event that is stressful for one person may not be for another.
3. Which specific organ is affected may in part be determined by early life experiences, but is also determined by constitutional, hereditary, or other factors which are unknown at this time.

We will briefly review the following proposals:

1. For every emotional state there is a specific physiologic concomitant which, if sustained, may, in the presence of other essential factors, lead to organ dysfunction and tissue damage (Alexander's theory[1]). Following a general review of this theory, we will present the application of it to peptic ulcer.

2. Reaction to stressful events, especially those involving loss or failure, may lead to an affective state of helplessness and hopelessness, which in turn has somatic consequences that influence the time of onset of disease. We will discuss this theory and its application to ulcerative colitis.

3. A number of investigations have resulted in empiric observations showing a correlation between psychosocial variables and incidence of organic disease. We will review two prospective studies that demonstrate a correlation between psychologic variables and the incidence of various disorders.

4. Evidence that glandular and visceral responses can be influenced by operant conditioning opens up the possibility that learning experiences may result in predisposition to psychosomatic disease, and that some symptoms may be learned or reinforced visceral responses. Miller[7] has pioneered investigations in this area and, in the laboratory animal, has demonstrated the effect of operant conditioning (instrumental learning) on salivation, intestinal contractions, heart rate, blood pressure, rate of urine formation, and other functions. His observations on the learning of visceral responses have led him to dispute the distinction made by Alexander and others between conversion symptoms mediated by the cerebrospinal nervous system and psychophysiologic symptoms mediated by the autonomic nervous system.[7] In addition to laboratory work with animals, clinical studies on humans have also demonstrated the effect of conditioning on visceral function, such as alteration of ventricular rate in patients with atrial fibrillation.[3]

While the application of learning theory to the study of psychosomatic disorders is promising, it should be noted that symptomatic response to learning, such as the alteration of ventricular rate in patients with atrial fibrillation associated with rheumatic heart disease, obviously does not imply that the development of the underlying disease was caused by conditioning experiences.

For further discussion of this important subject, the reader is referred to the reference section at the end of this chapter.

ALEXANDER'S THEORY

Preparatory to the elaboration of his own concepts, Alexander[1] cleared away much confusion by emphasizing that hysteric conversion symptoms involve "voluntary innervation, expressive movement, or sensory perceptions" and therefore can symbolically represent unconscious psychologic content. In contrast, while the viscera under autonomic nervous system influence do respond physiologically to emotional states, these responses do not represent direct, symbolic expression of unconscious feelings and ideas, although secondarily they may acquire symbolic significance.

283

Alexander believed that for every emotion there is a specific syndrome of physical changes and that when the emotion subsides the physiologic processes, such as those affecting heart rate and blood pressure, return to their baseline levels. However, if the emotion, such as fear, anger, or longing, cannot be expressed and relieved freely through voluntary activities but is repressed, the physiologic effects (mediated largely through the autonomic and neuroendocrine systems) are sustained, leading to chronic functional disturbance and eventually tissue damage. The disturbances of "vegetative functions" are divided into two categories corresponding to the emotional attitudes involved in (1) emergency preparations for fight or flight (predominantly sympathetic), or (2) withdrawal from outwardly directed activity (predominantly parasympathetic). If autonomic activation of either type is not followed by appropriate action, a chronic state of physiologic response persists followed by functional disorder or disease.

Alexander suggested that emotions of anger or aggression were associated with sympathetic stimulation and that blocking of aggressive or competitive behavior could eventually contribute to the development of a variety of disorders such as hypertension, migraine, hyperthyroidism, arthritis, vasodepressor syncope, and possibly diabetes. On the other hand, passive-dependent longings were associated with parasympathetic activity and if need-satisfying behaviors were blocked such disorders as peptic ulcer, constipation, diarrhea, colitis, and asthma might develop in some people. Alexander was careful to point out that various factors, other than psychologic, were also necessary in the production of these diseases, since many persons who develop conflicts involving aggression or passive longings do not become physically ill.

We will now consider some of the evidence concerning Alexander's concept of psychologic factors in peptic ulcer.

Peptic (Duodenal) Ulcer   Intensive study of individuals with peptic ulcer led Alexander and others to the conclusion that what characterized these patients was the presence of a conflict situation in which the patient wished to be dependent, loved, and cared for and in which these wishes were unfulfilled, either because the individual himself repudiated or repressed them or because of frustrating external circumstances. Noting that being loved and being fed are intimately associated from birth on, Alexander postulated that a frustrated, persistent longing for infantile dependence is associated with gastric hypersecretion, as if the individual is constantly preparing to be fed. The intensity of the conflict depends in part on external events. Severe sustained conflict eventually results in gastric dysfunction and peptic ulcer in some individuals.

This concept led to a now classic study of army inductees by Weiner et al,[14] in which they hypothesized that three factors contribute to development of duodenal ulcer: (1) sustained gastric hypersecretion (as reflected in high serum pepsinogen levels), (2) presence of the psychic conflict described above, and (3) exposure to an environmental event (induction into army) that mobilizes the conflict and induces psychic tension.[14] The subjects of their study were 2073 young men who were drafted into the army, for each of whom serum pepsinogen level was determined. Sixty-three subjects with values in the upper 15 percent and 57 with values in the lower 9 percent of serum pepsinogen level were selected for special study. Psychologic data were independently obtained and gastrointestinal x-ray examinations were done initially and later in basic training. Three subjects had healed duodenal ulcers and six subjects had active duodenal ulcers; all nine of these subjects were in the upper 15 percent of blood pepsinogen distribution. The psychologic data revealed that evidence of strong dependency needs was positively correlated with high pepsinogen levels. On the basis of the psychologic data, ten men (of 120) were selected as most likely to develop an ulcer; the predictions were accurate in seven out of the ten.

While the results of this study are compatible with predictions based on Alexander's theory, they nonetheless do not prove the theory. There is evidence that the characteristic of high serum pepsinogen levels tends to be present from very early in life and to persist throughout life. This observation raises the interesting possibility that infants with this characteristic may have unusually strong oral or nursing needs which, in turn, could predispose the individual to the kind of oral dependence conflict described by Alexander. Likelihood of the latter outcome would be enhanced if the infant with strong nursing needs happens to have a mother whose nursing capacity is limited.[5] It may also be noted that the above-cited investigation did not include a control group which was not exposed to the stress of induction into the army. Therefore this study does not shed light on how psychologic stress might affect gastroduodenal physiology in a way which leads to ulcer formation.

THE HELPLESSNESS–HOPELESSNESS THEORY

Many investigators have noted the frequency with which experiences involving separation from important other people or other kinds of important losses or disappointments are observed in close temporal connection with the onset or exacerbation of a wide variety of diseases. Engel and his co-workers at Strong Memorial Hospital, Rochester, New York, have been particularly active in clinical investigations designed to test the validity of this observation and in the development of a related theoretical conception of disease. The Rochester studies have included patients with ulcerative colitis, leukemia, lymphoma, and patients consecutively admitted to a medical inpatient service who were suffering from a variety of disorders. In 80 percent or more of patients interviewed, it was ascertained that an experience of loss or threatened loss had occurred shortly before the onset of illness or its exacerbation. Further, the experience of loss was interpreted as being highly significant to the patient in that it appeared to be followed by an affective state of helplessness and hopelessness.

Helplessness refers to a feeling of being deprived of an essential gratification as a result of a change in a relationship about which the patient feels powerless, so that his only recourse is to wait for a return of that which he has lost. Hopelessness refers to a feeling of despair or futility resulting from a loss of satisfaction for which the patient assumes complete responsibility and about which he can do nothing. Schmale and Engel refer to the inability to let go of wished for gratifications or unachievable goals as the "giving-up complex."[12] They interpret their data as indicating that, in some way, the giving-up complex acts as a permissive setting for factors present in the patient which predispose him to a particular somatic or psychic disorder, ie, as "a final common pathway to changes in health."[12]

The scientific establishment of this important concept is fraught with methodologic problems such as the difficulty in operationally defining the giving-up complex and in setting up blind, controlled studies. Indirect support for this theory has been obtained from studies of large groups of people in whom it was observed that morbidity and mortality rates are positively correlated with antecedent stress including that of bereavement.

We will now review the application of this theory to a specific disease, ulcerative colitis.

Ulcerative Colitis   In a series of papers published in the 1950s, Engel[4] reviewed the psychosomatic hypotheses of ulcerative colitis, certain somatic aspects of the disease, and reported observations on 39 of his own patients.

Many patients with ulcerative colitis have premorbid obsessive–compulsive character traits, tending to be neat, orderly, conscientious, stubborn. They frequently seem immature and tend to develop an ambivalent, dependent relationship with one or two persons who appear to be key figures in their lives. Except for these dependent relationships, these patients often appear to lack the capacity for close, warm friendships.

Onset of the illness and exacerbations were observed to be associated with a disturbance in the relationship with a key person in the patient's life and with the development of helplessness or despair. Further, Engel found that the ulcerative colitis patient had a history of a symbiotic relationship with his mother which left the patient permanently dependent on her or on a substitute, and that this accounts in part for the patient's vulnerability to separation. The question of why the patient becomes afflicted specifically with ulcerative colitis remains unanswered. It is clear that somatic factors, in addition to psychologic ones, are necessary for the development of the disease.

A Study of Precursors of Premature Disease and Death Thomas and her co-workers[13] have collected data bearing on a wide range of characteristics of a cohort of medical students prior to graduation from 17 successive classes beginning in 1948. In this continuing study, the subjects (now mostly physicians aged 35 to 55) have been followed and data pertaining to their health and that of their parents have been systematically obtained at regular intervals. The investigators have thus been able to compare the youthful characteristics of those subjects who have thus far remained in good health with those who have been affected by five disorders, namely, suicide, cancer, hypertension, myocardial infarction, and mental illness, the latter being defined as an emotional illness necessitating hospitalization.

Psychologic data were obtained from 1046 white male medical students. (Female subjects and subjects of other races were not included in the present analysis.) As of 1976, 109 of these subjects developed one of the above-listed disorders, as follows: 10 suicide, 30 mental illness, 34 cancer, 12 myocardial infarction, and 23 hypertension. The investigators compared psychologic data of one disorder group with that of another, and the disorder groups, separately and collectively, with a healthy control group matched for age, sex, and race.

Utilizing the Habits of Nervous Tension (HNT) Questionnaire, a checklist of 25 reactions to stressful situations, Thomas found that the mean HNT score of the total disorder group was significantly higher than that of the total control group. The highest mean scores were obtained by the suicide and mental illness groups; the mean scores of the cancer and hypertension groups were close to the score of the control group. Scores on an HNT subscale relating to anxiety were higher for four of the disorder groups—suicide, mental illness, myocardial infarction, and hypertension—than for the control group, whereas the score for the cancer group was slightly lower than that of the total control group. Responses to a Family Attitude Questionnaire indicate that the suicide, mental illness, and cancer groups may have had an unusual lack of closeness to their parents when the questionnaire was administered to them as medical students. The finding that students who were later to develop cancer felt alienated from their parents was unexpected by the investigators.

Thomas is properly cautious in interpreting these and other correlations noted between psychologic characteristics observed in youth and the subsequent development of physical and emotional disorders. Thus, she notes that association between two variables does not necessarily mean that one (the antecedent variable) caused the other. Engel comments that Thomas's work provides major support for the postulate, based on retrospective studies, that people with different disease predisposition also may differ in psychologic characteristics.[6]

Coronary Heart Disease (CHD)   Near the turn of the century, Osler reported his impressions that heredity, rich diet, and psychologic stress contributed to the etiology of atherosclerosis. He also commented that the typical patient with coronary disease is a "keen and ambitious man, the indicator of whose engines is always set 'full speed ahead.' "[8] In subsequent years, a number of clinical observers have reported similar observations.

Not until the work of Rosenman et al was the accuracy of these clinical impressions tested by a controlled, blind, prospective study.[10] These investigators predicted that individuals who showed evidence of "behavior pattern type A" would have a higher incidence of CHD than would persons who did not. Type A behavior pattern is characterized by excessive drive, aggressiveness, ambition, an enhanced sense of time urgency, and relatively great preoccupation with competitive activity, deadlines, and similar pressures. By means of an oral questionnaire, 3182 male subjects who were free of evidence of CHD were classified as exhibiting behavior pattern type A or as not exhibiting that pattern (type B). Numerous other data were obtained at the outset of the study including socioeconomic data, smoking habits, and physiologic and biochemical measures. During a two-year follow-up the subjects were reevaluated for evidence of CHD by a senior medical referee who was independent of the study. During the two-year period, 54 cases of CHD developed among the 1584 subjects exhibiting pattern A, as compared with 16 cases among the 1598 subjects exhibiting pattern B. For the group as a whole, the relative risk ratio, type A/type B, was 3.40; among younger subjects (age 39 to 49 years) the relative risk ratio was 6.48, compared with 1.88 in older subjects (age 50 to 59 years).

Other studies have, in addition, provided evidence that the incidence of life stresses is positively correlated with subsequent development of CHD and with elevation of blood cholesterol, acceleration of blood clotting, and stimulation of the autonomic nervous system.[11]

IMPLICATIONS FOR MANAGEMENT

Comprehensive management of patients with psychosomatic diseases rests upon an understanding of the pathophysiology of the disorders and upon a grasp of psychologic factors which may have contributed to the development of illness. It is apparent that if psychologic problems have contributed to the onset of an illness, their persistence or recurrence may impede recovery or contribute to relapse. In most cases of psychosomatic disease, the psychologic aspects of management can best be incorporated into the total treatment approach by the primary physician. In selected cases, the physician may find psychiatric consultation useful and occasionally he may choose to refer the patient to a psychiatrist for psychotherapy.

In the paragraphs below, we will briefly discuss only the psychologic aspects of management of patients with peptic ulcer, ulcerative colitis, and coronary heart disease. The psychologic principles of management of these disorders logically follow from an understanding of the emotional factors associated with them.

Peptic Ulcer   In the management of peptic ulcer, it is important to (1) ascertain what kind of stress, if any, was associated with the onset or current exacerbation of the disease, and (2) attempt to provide the patient with satisfaction of his dependency needs in a manner acceptable to him. If, for example, the precipitating stress involved dependency need –deprivation secondary to marital conflict, it will be necessary to help the patient cope with the marital problems. This may involve the physician in working directly with the spouse as well as the patient. In addition, the physician himself can provide acceptable means of dependency gratification by establishing a relationship that evokes a sense of security in the patient, by scheduling return visits, by prescribing periods of rest or vacations, and by careful attention to symptom alleviation through dietary and drug treatment.

Ulcerative Colitis   In this serious, sometimes life-threatening disorder, the role of the physician in instituting medical and/or surgical procedures of crucial importance to the patient's life results in the physician becoming a person of profound significance to the patient. That is, the patient–physician relationship itself may become the key relationship upon which the patient comes to depend. This is particularly apt to occur if the illness episode was precipitated by the loss of an important person in the patient's life. As is true of other important, dependent relationships in his life, the patient is apt eventually to exhibit evidence of ambivalent feelings toward the physician. The ambivalence may be manifested in many ways, such as exhibiting mistrust or occasionally by testing the physician's competence or commitment to the patient's care.

It is important that the physician's relationship with the patient be a stable one. The physician should guard against being provoked by ambivalent behavior. The impact of separations from the patient can be lessened by explaining their necessity and duration to the patient and sometimes by giving him a prescription to keep and use as needed. As rapport is established, the patient is encouraged to discuss his life situation and to express feelings. Referral to the psychiatrist for consultation or psychotherapy may be indicated, but should be done in such a way that the patient feels it to be an addition to his therapeutic regimen, not a substitute for his relationship with the primary physician.

Coronary Heart Disease   We will confine our discussion to patients with myocardial infarction. In the first two or three days of the acute illness, virtually all patients are apprehensive, some severely so. Frequent contact with the patient, reassurance both explicit and implied by an attitude of confidence and optimism, and administration of a minor tranquilizer may be indicated. If the patient exhibits denial of his illness, it is generally wise not to disturb this defense unless the denial leads to behavior that seriously compromises treatment. It may be helpful to assess the patient's need to comprehend his condition and accordingly to give him an understandable explanation of his illness.

After the first two or three days, the patient may become depressed. This may occur in any patient with an acute myocardial infarction, but is perhaps particularly frequent and severe in individuals who have a history of type A behavior. These patients may find the temporary immobilization necessitated by treatment very difficult to bear and, in some cases, it is wise to liberalize the treatment plan to allow the patient somewhat more mobility than is ordinarily done. The patient's depression may be related to his anticipation of not being able to return to his customary high level of activity. This should be discussed with the patient. Some patients exaggerate the degree of disability they face and need to be given a more realistic appraisal of their prospects for returning to a useful life.

When the patient's condition becomes stable, physical rehabilitation through carefully graded passive and active exercises is begun and is continued following discharge from the hospital.

The patient, particularly if he has exhibited type A behavior characteristics, will need help in learning to modify his life style. He will need much support and guidance in learning how to relax, to give himself rest periods, to keep his ambitions from ceaselessly driving him, and to learn to take his time in the accomplishment of tasks. This educative effort will require persistence and patience on the part of the physician, the family, and the patient himself.

REFERENCES

1. Alexander F: Psychosomatic Medicine. New York, Norton, 1950
2. Bard P: A diencephalic mechanism for the expression of rage with special references to the sympathetic nervous system. Am J Physiol 84:490, 1928
3. Bleecker ER, Engel BT: Learned control of ventricular rate in patients with atrial fibrillation. Psychosom Med 35:161, 1973
4. Engel GL: Studies of ulcerative colitis. III. The nature of the psychologic processes. Am J Med 19:231, 1955
5. Engel GL: Psychophysiological gastrointestinal disorders. 1. Peptic ulcer. In Freedman AM, Kaplan HI, Sadock BJ (eds): Comprehensive Textbook of Psychiatry, 2nd ed. Baltimore, Williams and Wilkins, 1975, Chap 26.3
6. Engel GL: The predictive value of psychological variables for disease and death. Ann Intern Med 85:673, 1976

7. Miller NE: Learning of visceral and glandular responses. Science 163:434, 1969
8. Osler W: Lectures on angina pectoris and allied states. New York Med J 4:224, 1896
9. Pincus JH, Tucker GJ: Behavioral Neurology. New York, Oxford Univ Press, 1974
10. Rosenman RH, Friedman M, Straus R, et al: Coronary heart disease in the western collaborative study group. JAMA 195:130, 1966
11. Russek HI: Role of emotional stress in the etiology of clinical coronary heart disease. Dis Chest 52:1, 1967
12. Schmale AH: Giving up as a final common pathway to changes in health. Adv Psychosom Med 8:20, 1972
13. Thomas CB: Precursors of premature disease and death. Ann Intern Med 85:653, 1976
14. Weiner H, Thaler M, Reiser MF, Mirsky IA: Etiology of duodenal ulcer. Psychosom Med 19:1, 1957

Index